GIFTED
INTELLIGENCE

Anne Angelone

ANNE ANGELONE

Copyright © by Anne Angelone 2018

All Rights Reserved

ISBN-13: 978-1726340779
ISBN-10: 1726340775

No part of this publication may be reproduced in any form or by any means, including scanning, photocopying, or otherwise without prior written permission of the copyright holder. Image Credit: with permission from canva.com

Disclaimer: This guide is not intended to provide medical advice or to take the place of medical advice and treatment from your personal physician. Readers are advised to consult their own doctors or other qualified health professionals regarding the treatment of medical conditions.

The author shall not be held liable or responsible for any misunderstanding or misuse of the information contained in this manual or for any loss, damage, or injury caused or alleged to be caused directly or indirectly by any treatment, action, or application of any food or food source discussed in this program manual. The information in this guide has not been evaluated by the U.S. Food and Drug Administration. This information is not intended to diagnose, treat, cure, or prevent any disease. To request permission for reproduction, please contact:

Website: www.anneangelone.com

Table of Contents

Introduction 5

Gifted Personality Traits 7

The Hyper-Brain, Hyper-Body Theory 10

Neurobiological Approach 12

Asynchronous Development 13

The Two Hemispheres 15

Personality Neuroscience 18

The Human Connectome 19

Brain Networks 20

Dominant Neural Networks and the 5 Q Model of
   Gifted Intelligence 23

Cognitive Brain Maps 25

Emotional Brain Maps 30

Intellectual Overexcitabilities 33

Emotional Overexcitabilities 37

Imaginational Overexcitabilities 40

Sensual Overexcitabilities 45

Psychomotor Overexcitabilities 68

Humanistic Psychology 80

Final Thoughts 118

"We often speak about the benefits of being in nature…and then I remember, we are in nature – our bodies *are* nature."

~Swami Ramananda

Introduction

As autoimmune, mood, sensory, learning and behavioral problems continue to explode into the health arena, identifying the way stress and chronic inflammation exacerbate these issues will become the most important trending topic of research in the years to come. A little-known fact is that many of these problems are related to gifted intelligence. The term *gifted* refers to an ability to sense, perceive and interpret the world in a quicker and more detailed manner than the bulk of the population.

As we start to identify the sensory, cognitive, psychomotor and emotional imprints that underlie these issues, it becomes apparent that the number one hidden issue driving our chronic diagnoses may be unrecognized gifted intelligences. That is, most of these issues may be traced back to one or more areas of the brain that are considered "hot spots" or highly charged neural circuits that present as gifted personality traits. We can see our gifted traits manifesting as sensory, immunologic, learning, behavior and psycho-emotional issues especially when we are stressed and inflamed.

If you are unaware of your gifted intelligence and lack the knowledge of how to cool these hot spots (before they become overactive), you may be living with the effect of undue flare-ups. Highly charged neural circuits may express phenotypically as psychobiological symptoms (such as depression) but may then proceed toward neurodegeneration due to environmental inputs, stress, and level of inflammation. At whatever stage, symptoms indicate clues to brain areas that need rehabilitation or improved functional connectivity.

As we shall see, whether the diagnosis is autoimmune disease, autism spectrum disorder (ASD), anxiety, depression, OCD or ADHD, we can look at all of these as brain circuits that progress according to the degree of stress, inflammation and comorbidities that present for each person. Instead of seeing all of these as disorders or diseases, we could look at them more as emotional/social, behavioral, learning and/or sensory-motor challenges. At the end of the day, we can see that they are all disorders of cognitive, sensory, motor and emotional regulation. In essence, it's generally about a hypo or hyper functioning prefrontal cortex that can neither regulate the immune system nor integrate sensory and emotional triggers.

Gifted intelligence explores the psycho-neuro-immuno-sensory-motor forces that predispose us to mood, sensory, learning, behavioral and autoimmune disorders. In this book, you will learn why all of these so-called diseases and disorders can and should be treated as learning opportunities. Integrating existing constructs from behavior theory, cognitive neuroscience, functional neurology, humanistic psychology and emerging yoga and meditation research, this book is intended to guide future clinical research, specifically targeting areas of development in the treatment of immune, affective, sensory and self-regulation disorders.

Neuroscience tells us that we can actually change the brain with consistent effort. This is called neuroplasticity. We are discovering that, despite genetics, the brain can be rewired specifically with neuroplastic techniques. I will outline solid neuroplastic strategies to support the gifted brain. The goal is to identify and use our gifted intelligences wisely.

Gifted Personality Traits

Gifted individuals see, hear, sense, feel, think and imagine to a degree that is foreign to many others. They are highly empathic and use their refined perceptions to innovate and create – getting endlessly absorbed in art, logic, athletics, writing and/or music.

Most people think that giftedness only pertains to advanced intellectual abilities. However, giftedness is actually a mosaic of personality traits that go beyond IQ tests. In addition to high intelligence, other qualities of giftedness include sensitivity, perfectionism, entelechy (the ability to intuit and manifest impulses), introversion and the "autonomous factor," which is when someone is not interested in other's opinions about the things they create that are important to them.

Intellectual drive, movement, imagination, sensation, creativity, and a deep sense of justice and empathy are all great things, but the fallout may show up as allergies, anxiety, depression, ADHD, increased environmental sensitivities and autoimmune reactions. Unless these traits are recognized, it can greatly impact one's quality of life.

Dabrowski's concept of overexcitabilities (OEs) can help us understand giftedness. In the 1920's, Kazimierz Dabrowski, a Polish psychiatrist, developed the Theory of Positive Disintegration, which proposes a high potential for personal development in people who have overexcitabilities.

Dabrowski observed that some individuals have an innate ability to react more strongly than others and used the term overexcitability (OE) to describe this trait. According to Dabrowski, bright individuals tended to be "neurotically allergic or nervous" (Liebowitz, 2017). They demonstrated a uniquely heightened way of experiencing and responding to their environment within five specific areas: psychomotor, sensual, intellectual, imaginational, and emotional domains, which he referred to as overexitabilities. He found these overexcitabilities to be associated with personality development and observed symptoms of slight neuroses among them as well, such as depression, mild anxiety, and tics (Mendaglio, 2008).

The nervous systems of people with OEs are more sensitive and responsive to stimuli. Dabrowski believed that the stronger the overexcitability, the more intense the inner conflict and frustration an individual might experience. He believed that gifted people struggle in the gap between their current self and their personality ideal. This gap can be seen as a key area for personality growth and healing. For the gifted, inner conflict is considered a developmental rather than a degenerative sign, because it encourages the person to replace current ways of living with those of higher level development.

So, gifted people who have big reactions to stimuli and higher levels of emotional and/or sensory distress should know that advancing into higher levels of development is predicated on seeing and understanding overexcitabilities as holding developmental potential for individuation and autonomy.

Overexcitabilities should be embraced as a key part of human developmental and life experience. We can look at symptoms as a having something important to tell us and not as mental, emotional, or physical illnesses. Instead, symptoms can be a road map to a more evolved self. We can see how challenges can be a positive sign in that they lead us to a deeper understanding of what is happening at a brain-based level.

In this way, our current negative view of mental health, immune, sensory, and/or learning and behavioral issues will be reframed. We can look at all aspects of gifted intelligence as a means to know a person's preferences and also their weaknesses. Drawing on this theory, I have evolved the concept of overexcitabilities as dominant neural networks.

In this book, I describe overexcitabilities as dominant neural networks that may or may not be functionally connected. As a result, they may be hyper or hypofunctional and lead to issues with sensory-motor, emotional, intuitive and/or cognitive challenges. The task is improving dysfunctional neural networks with neuroplastic techniques, along with whole brain balancing for areas that need support.

The aim of this book is to increase knowledge and understanding of how to be in charge of our cognition, senses, emotions and behavior so as to cut off potential downstream reactions that biology/genetics may have in store for us. When we learn more about the brain networks involved, we can be more responsible for and responsive to the sensory input, thoughts and emotions that drive our behaviors and immune responses.

Knowing the map circuitry and having the right tools to improve functional connectivity in our brain and body will be explored through a process of psycho-neuro-sensory-immuno-behavioral awareness and integration. Methods to support functional connectivity will be introduced to regulate all cortices and networks of the brain. With more integration and hemispheric balance, we can even out our overexcitabilities and support overall brain connectivity.

ANNE ANGELONE

The Hyper-Brain, Hyper-Body Theory

Very few studies have investigated the psycho-neuro-immunological (PNI) interplay between intelligence and affective, autoimmune, sensory, learning, and behavioral disorders. However, one recent study queried whether there is a link between a heightened cognitive capacity (hyper-brain) and heightened psychological and subsequent physiological immune responses (hyper-body) (Karpinski et al., 2017).

Researchers examined the prevalence of mood and anxiety disorders, ADHD, food and environmental sensitivities, allergies, asthma, autoimmune disease, and ASD in 3,715 participants (at or above the ninety-eighth percentile of intelligence) and found evidence to support their hyper-brain, hyper-body hypothesis. Part of the study sought to discover if those with high intelligence also had signs of OEs as described by Dabrowski.

They first noticed that overexcitabilities tended to be diagnosed along with food and environmental sensitivities, anxiety, depression, ASD, ADHD and/or autoimmune disease, and sought to discover if those with OEs led to "bigger" expression and intensity of symptoms and if anxiety, depression and rumination were also driving the expression of autoimmune reactions in a vicious cycle. Interestingly, they found that high intellectual capacity is a risk factor for each of the above psychological and physiological conditions and that a combination of emotional, imaginational, and sensual overexcitabilities were associated with all of these presentations.

That is, they noticed that those with a high intellectual capacity (hyper-brain) possessed a combination of overexcitabilities (sensual, imaginational, and emotional) that may predispose them to anxiety, depression, ADHD, OCD as well as physiological conditions involving elevated sensory and altered immune and inflammatory responses including ASD, food and environmental sensitivities, allergies and autoimmune disease (hyper-body).

Since overexcitabilities tended to be diagnosed along with allergies, food and environmental sensitivities, anxiety, depression, OCD, ASD, ADHD and/or autoimmune disease, we need to consider the underlying dominant neural circuits that lead to bigger expression and intensity of symptoms.

Neurobiological Approach

We need a comprehensive way of understanding gifted people who present with autoimmune, mood, sensory, learning and behavioral issues. We need to question whether gifted personality traits may be driving the polarity of the immune system and creating unnecessary flare-ups. We need to do this not to pathologize gifted tendencies, but to understand gifted individuals better and bring balance in a simple and practical way. When we get curious about the overlapping biological basis of many of the neurobehavioral, psychological and neuropsychiatric diseases, we see how the neurobiological structures in the brain may be dysfunctionally or aberrantly connected.

To investigate this, we need to unpack the sensory, psychomotor, emotional, intuitive and cognitive processes of the individual. We need to know what neuro-circuits are being activated when gifted modes launch, and how to keep them balanced. We need to take great care around gifted intelligences and know how to use them wisely as power tools for personal growth. We need to acknowledge all of the intelligences embedded in those who suffer from being exposed to an environmentally and socially toxic world. We need to identify and temper chaotic experiences of the environment to be able to protect ourselves in ways that feel congruent with the psyche.

Asynchronous Development

Giftedness also refers to 'asynchronous development.' Asynchrony happens when the rate of cognitive, emotional and motor development are out of sync. If the timing and rhythm is off in any part of the brain, emotional, sensory-motor, and immune imbalances will occur as a downstream effect. The remedy is to improve plasticity upstream where the issue is - in the brain.

This concept has been applied clinically by Functional Neurologists for learning about neurobehavioral issues such as ASD and ADHD, and can also be applied to those with sensory processing, affective and autoimmune disease, as they also represent a right brain imbalance. Think of the brain as being at a loss in terms of having a lack of adequate sensory, cognitive and emotional stimulation, processing and integration. This could lead to heightened sensitivity and emotional issues ranging from social inhibition and negative affect to anxiety and depression. These tendencies are all considered right brain deficits in specific processing centers, namely, the limbic, sensory and cognitive integration areas.

A Functional Neurologist would say that this lack of brain stimulation, processing, and integration is considered the primary problem in functionally disconnected brains, which shows up when learning, immune, sensory, emotional, social and behavioral dysfunctions occur, due to the fact that the brain is out of sync. I believe it is responsible for many of the physical, mental, emotional and social difficulties related to the whole spectrum of neurobehavioral (ADHD), neuropsychological (anxiety/depression) and neurobiological disorders, including autoimmune disease.

Having a brain-based understanding of cognitive, psychomotor, sensory, emotional and resultant immunological patterns gives us knowledge that we can do something about. At the end of the day, correcting autoimmune, mood, sensory processing, learning and behavior will rely on improving right hemispheric function by giving it the correct inputs that it has been lacking.

The first thing we need to understand is that the brain can be supported and rewired. With new sensory-motor inputs (including specific exercises, sound therapies, music, essential oils) we can change the brain. This is called neuroplasticity, which refers to the fact that the brain can change both physically and chemically in response to specific kinds of activity.

Fixing neurobiological deficits with neuroplastic exercises is called functional integration. Neuroplastic exercises may include acupuncture, yoga postures, music, sound, essential oil therapy and proprioceptive exercises.

What needs to be addressed are any areas of imbalance that can be causing both psychological and/or immune dysfunction. We can change the strength and number of neural connections with precise stimulation to areas that need it most. For example, if we know that the neurobiological blueprint of fear behaviors is based in the amygdala, with poor prefrontal control, we can work on improving top-down control of the prefrontal cortex (PFC) to regulate the amygdala. We can also consider subcortical supports such as essential oil therapy to calm the amygdala. Now let's look at the main brain areas involved in functional integration and hemispheric balance.

The Two Hemispheres

Even though there is no physical difference between the right and left hemispheres of the brain, the way they perceive and process information is different. The brain is not genetically programmed to become right or left, rather it becomes right and left because of experience and stimulation that it is exposed to in the environment.

The left hemisphere is in charge of the motor system and is conditioned by exercise and balance. The right hemisphere controls cognitive, sensory and emotional integration and is conditioned by environmental inputs and by getting our neurobiological needs met, i.e., for safety, reward and belonging. At the most basic level, we are a walking nervous and immune system that is governed by the laws of nature/nurture affecting us via the senses.

The Left Hemisphere
Think of the left hemisphere as reflecting both the motor system and initial approach behavior. Approach behavior is reflected down to the cellular level as the motor nerves follow the interpretation of felt-sense information from internal or external cues. When approaching a situation, the body is taking in all sorts of sensory information and the emotional system (related to the right hemisphere) is hopefully giving us accurate clues about whether or not it is safe to continue.

The left hemisphere is in charge of logic, language and literalness (Siegel & Hartzell, 2003). That is, the left hemisphere is the side that makes sense of our experiences in definable words that give meaning and order to our chaotic emotional and sensory inputs. The neocortex on the left side is actually wired to support this sense of order, placing information into neat packets that give the sensation of a yes/no and right/wrong binary system (Hawkins & Blakeslee, 2004).

Learning Disorders

Learning disorders reflect a lack of functional connectivity in brain areas that process and communicate information. Learning challenges can present with varying degrees of severity, and some people may struggle with more than one. As the human population lives longer, the aging brain may manifest with the same learning challenges that usually present in childhood. By understanding these challenges and the brain areas involved, we can add in the necessary supports for the brain to be as healthy as it can be on any given day.

Since the left hemisphere controls reading speed and accuracy, math calculations, language skills, motor coordination and writing skills, we need to support the left brain to improve these functions. Not surprisingly, the remedy for all learning challenges (whether neurodevelopmental or neurodegenerative) includes sensory-motor and brain game activities to improve functional connectivity for processing and learning. Sensory-motor activities improve rhythm and timing, which also leads to optimal brain-body-immune balance, muscle tone, learning and emotional regulation. The upshot is that the brain, even when asynchronous, can be improved by targeting deficient areas.

The Right Hemisphere

The right hemisphere puts the brakes on the immune system, controls avoidance behavior and autonomic responses, governs proprioception, reading of emotions, facial expression, tone of voice, and the insular cortex. The insular cortex is a key component of the salience network, which we use to integrate cognitive, sensory and emotional information. A weakness in any of these areas signals a right brain weakness.

Right hemisphere processing is nonlinear, taking everything in at once in a receptive way (Siegel et al., 2003). The right hemisphere is also specialized for perceiving and processing visual and spatial information. This includes sending and receiving nonverbal signals, the key to social understanding.

Right brain weaknesses can manifest as awkward social behavior, ADHD, OCD, sensory processing issues, allergies, food and environmental sensitivities, anxiety/depression, eczema, asthma, brain fog, leaky gut and autoimmune disease. All of these basically result from a combination of genetics, environmental insults, skin, lung, gut, and brain barrier system dysfunctions along with a lack of sensory, cognitive and emotional regulation. The problem with untreated right brain deficiency is that the leaky gut, food sensitivities, mood swings, social problems and autoimmune disease will continue.

However, if we investigate giftedness through the lens of neurobiology, we come to understand that the right hemisphere of the brain is in need of support. In essence, we are still looking down stream when we should be looking upstream where the issue is, which is in the brain. If an individual's emotional/social/immune and or sensory-motor difficulties are showing up, we need to look no further than right hemisphere deficiency. So, we can get rid of all the names of the disorders, all the names of the diseases, and look at the expression to clue us in to the areas that need support. We also need to learn how to retool the brain with neuroplastic props and *learn* some key principles from modern neuroscience.

Personality Neuroscience

Although we traditionally have been taught to study personality at a biological trait level, we now know that the brain is the source of all human behavior. In recent years, the neurobiological substrates of personality have been explored by looking at brain structure and function, which is considered the premier backdrop of behavioral expression. Identifying the neural mechanisms that underlie differences in personality, along with environmental and cultural influences, has been the focus of the emerging field of personality neuroscience.

The time has arrived for us to be considering gifted personality traits (in terms of learning, sensory processing, affective disorders and autoimmune disease) in a completely different way. Borrowing the latest ideas from neuroscience and bringing them into clinical practice has so far been the work of Functional Neurologists. The goal now is to apply what we know from neuroscience to neuropsychiatric, neurobehavioral, sensory processing disorders and autoimmune disease. The treatment is geared toward rehabilitating the right or left-brain imbalances that cause the expression in the first place.

Now that we have covered the right and left hemispheres, let's continue with a basic understanding of the human connectome.

The Human Connectome

Healthy brain function requires effective integration of neural information between distributed brain regions. This is supported by white matter axonal projections of the brain, which together form a complex network that is known as the human connectome. This neural network has been proposed to give rise to and shape the collective and coordinated neural phenomena underlying cognitive processes (Van Den Heuval, 2011). Studies have linked connectome organization to general intelligence, working memory performance, executive functioning, personality and even creativity (Ryman et al., 2014).

From the point of view of the aging brain, we need to energize these parts of the brain to maintain plasticity. It really is the use it or lose it model. However, in the case of the gifted, we may need to learn how to relax our brains because such high synchrony of certain brain networks may lead to some of our problem symptoms and behaviors.

Brain Networks

In order to attain optimal brain function, we first need to understand our repertoire of brain states and how to shift them as needed. This can help us facilitate change not only emotionally and mentally but also behaviorally. What follows is a brief description of the predominant brain networks that we typically function with in our lifetimes.

THE TOP 3 BRAIN NETWORKS

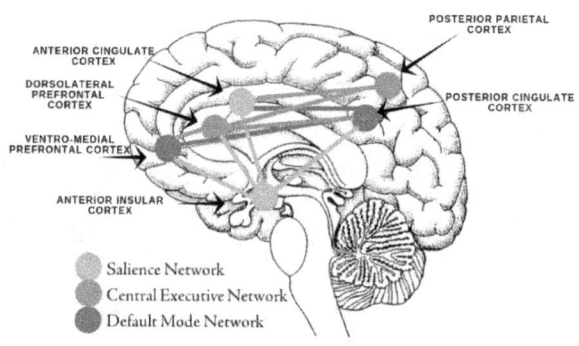

The Top 3 Networks

1. The central executive network (CEN) is used for sustained attention, working memory, and monitoring goal-directed behavior. The CEN is comprised of the dorsolateral prefrontal cortex (PFC) and the posterior parietal cortex (PPC) and activates when we need to focus or control our thought processes.

2. The Default Mode Network (DMN) is the brain network, which processes self-referencing information. The DMN includes the precuneus and the posterior cingulate cortex

(PCC), as well as more frontal regions like the ventro-medial frontal cortex (vmPFC) and the inferior parietal regions (Damoiseaux et al., 2006). The DMN is active when thoughts are directed towards internal processes like idea generation, mind wandering, daydreaming and imagining. The DMN deactivates during processing of external stimuli, e.g. cognitive tasks which activate the CEN instead.

3. The salience network (SN) is responsible for alternating between idea generation (DMN) and idea evaluation (CEN). The salience network includes two main nodes: the anterior cingulate cortex (ACC) and the anterior insular cortex (AIC). The insula is also involved in consciousness, perception, self-awareness, cognitive functioning, interpersonal experience, emotion and the regulation of the body's homeostasis. The ACC is involved with analyzing information, making it salient. In doing so, the ACC relies on the emotional centers to make this determination, and is involved in our sense of intuition. The ACC is also involved in self-referential tasks, theory of mind (ToM), detecting errors and monitoring conflict. The salience network also extends throughout the ventral tegmental area, substantia nigra, the amygdala and ventral striatum.

Other Important Networks

1. The Frontoparietal Control Network (FPCN) is used for intention setting, reappraisal and response inhibition. It is also associated with self-care, moral cognition and prosocial behavior.
2. The Dorsal Attention Network (DAN) helps with sustained attention.
3. The Cortico-Striato-Thalamo-Cortical (CSTC) pathway,

and more specifically, the Striato-Pallido-Thalamo-Cortical network (SPTCN) is responsible for extinction learning and optimal self-regulation (Gard, T. et al., 2014).
4. The hypothalamic–pituitary–adrenal (HPA) axis supports parasympathetic control and homeostasis across all systems.

Now let's consider the dominant neural networks related to gifted intelligence.

Dominant Neural Networks and the 5 Q Model of Gifted Intelligence

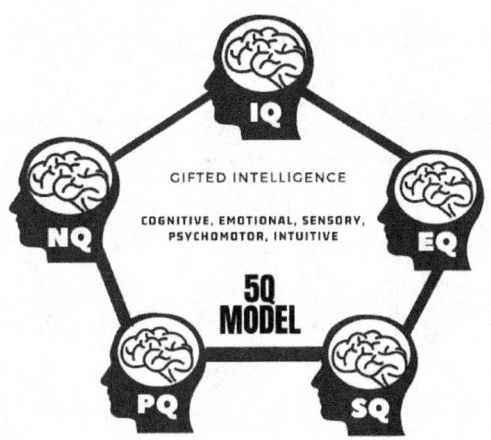

I use a convenient 5Q or 5 Intelligence model to describe how all aspects of our psychic nature – cognition, emotions, sensory, motor and intuitive experiences can be identified. Why Q? IQ traditionally refers to your intelligence quotient or IQ score. In this writing, I am looking into the amount of functional connectivity in brain networks as the backdrop of each intelligence. EQ refers to your emotional intelligence, SQ refers to your sensory intelligence, PQ to psychomotor intelligence and NQ refers to intuitive intelligence.

In the 5Q Intelligence model, each style of intelligence has a dominant neural net with varying levels of functional connectivity per person. This likely expresses as dominant tendencies in our personality. The other "intelligence networks" within our brain-body also have varying levels of functional connectivity and may express less than the dominant function. All intelligences are equally important and can help us learn a lot about ourselves and how to improve all aspects of our psychic (sensory-motor-intuitive-cognitive-emotional) self.

The ultimate goal of healing is to recover all part of ourselves. In the case of our psyche, we can view all of the intelligences as facets of our basic human drives that may be weak or strong in us – expressing too loudly or not loudly enough – and are always in flux with the environment. It's not just about balancing our dominant neural nets; it's also about learning what's required for congruent self-expression. This model will teach you how to support your dominant and non-dominant styles of sensing, moving, thinking, learning and feeling. This will make it easier to navigate and process the emotional, social and sensory world around you.

Cognitive Brain Maps

Having been inspired by Dario Nardi's work on Meyer's Briggs personality traits in his book, *The Neuroscience of Personality: Brain Savvy Insights for All Types of People*, I have evolved some of these concepts with the gifted 5Q model. In my model, I introduce dominant neural networks and include both cognitive (cortical) and emotional (limbic) maps for the gifted brain. Let's start with Cognitive Brain Maps.

To simplify and hone in on the areas of interest, I will use the 10-20 system, which is an internationally recognized method of locating scalp electrodes for an EEG exam. This system is a great way of peering into the underlying areas of the brain, specifically the cerebral cortex. The zones are numbered and labeled according to the corresponding lobes of the brain. O1 and O2 correlate to the occipital lobe zones; T3, T4, T5 and T6 are zones of the temporal lobe; P3 and P4 zones are located on the parietal lobe; C3 and C4 are associated with the central area of the brain; PF1 and PF2 zones match to the prefrontal cortex and finally, F3, F4, F7 and F8 are associated to the frontal cortex area. The associated functions of each area are derived from Brodmann maps of the brain. I will use these areas to describe the dominant neural networks for each kind of intelligence. Please note that while the 10-20 system uses FP1 and FP2 to denote the prefrontal region, I use the PF1 and PF2 for ease of reading the word prefrontal.

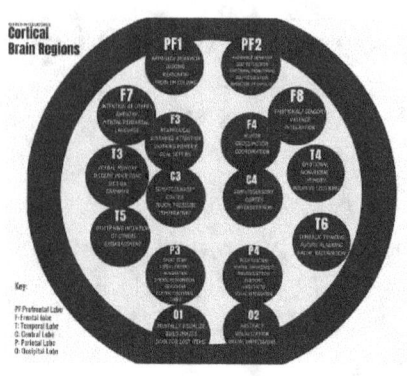

Brain Maps	Brain Region	Functions
	PF1	**Prefrontal Region # 1 = PF1** is involved in judging, evaluating and initiating approach behaviors, decision making, reasoning and analytic thinking. This region is also responsible for filtering negative information, noticing errors and providing reasons.
	PF2	**Prefrontal Region #2 = PF2** is used when a person is involved in self-reflection, emotional monitoring, self-regulation, avoidance behavior and inhibition of impulses.
	F3	**Frontal Region #3 = F3** is considered the seat of planning, sustained attention and working memory, i.e., the ability of the brain to hold information while processing it.
	F4	**Frontal Region #4 = F4** This area has to do with understanding humor, categorizing and defining. F4 is responsive to tactile stimuli, visual stimuli and auditory stimuli. This region is also involved with inhibition of responses, maintaining motor coordination, verbal reasoning and problem solving. This same part of the brain is also associated with

		social and emotional judgment and planning.
	F7	**Frontal Region #7 = F7** has a role in integrating sensory information. This area is considered part of the "frontal mirror neuron system" which helps us engage in mental rehearsal, verbal expression, mood regulation, anticipation of reward and assessing the intention of others. It also triggers empathy. Those with high emotional, intuitive and sensory intelligence likely have high activity in F7.
	F8	**Frontal Region #8 = F8** is also recruited for emotional regulation, social inhibition and emotional/personal values. Region F8 works in conjunction with PF01 to notice errors in values and restrain emotional reactions. F8 has to do with recall of details, modesty, personal beliefs and literal recall. F8 helps us with personal decisions, autobiographical memories, future goals and events. It is also the area that is stimulated when we rank things in order of importance or when we discuss our values. This coincides with our inner value system, cognitive and emotional valence.
	P3	**Parietal Region #3 = P3** is part of the mirror neuron system and is involved in copying emotional tones, innuendo, nuance and non-verbal memory. It also has to do with identifying objects, symbol recognition, rote math, reading, spelling, cognitive reasoning, attention, short-term memory, imagination and theory of mind (ToM).
	P4	**Parietal Region #4 = P4** is the site related to proprioception that allows us to sense ourselves in space. P4 is also involved in visuomotor control or

		directing attention as well as maintaining an alert state.
	O1	**Occipital Region #1 = O1** is where we mentally visualize and build images, and scan the environment for lost items.
	O2	**Occipital Region #2 = O2** has to do with abstract visualization and visual patterns. This region helps us gain an impression of an image, place or a person's character from appearance.
	T3	**Temporal Region #3 = T3** handles language, including verbal memory, phonological processing, diction, grammar and voice tone. T3 has to do with hearing words of self/others while T4 has to do with discerning tone of voice and weighing the motivation and intent of others. When humming, speaking and listening to music, T3 and T4 are recruited.
	T4	**Temporal Region #4 = T4** – this area supports intuitive listening. T4 also relates to emotional non-verbal memory.
	T5	**Temporal Region #5 = T5** is recruited when we are curious about someone's thinking, including being very aware of what they are not saying. T5 is also recruited when we feel embarrassed.
	T6	**Temporal Region #6 = T6** is used when we are making predictions, thinking symbolically and strategizing about the future. T6 also lends to emotional understanding, facial recognition and auditory processing. T5 and T6 are both involved in social feedback.
	C3	**Central Region #3 = C3 (and C4)** is located on the top of the primary somatosensory cortex. This part of our brain is responsible for processing touch

		and interoception as well as keeping track of the location of our body parts (proprioception) (De Boeck, 2010). This along with P4 gives us a sense of where we are in space, how we move in relation to other people and how things affect us physically.
	C4	**Central Region #4 =** C4 houses the somatosensory cortex, which integrates sensory information, including interoception, touch, pressure, temperature, pain and spatial awareness (proprioception).

Emotional Brain Maps

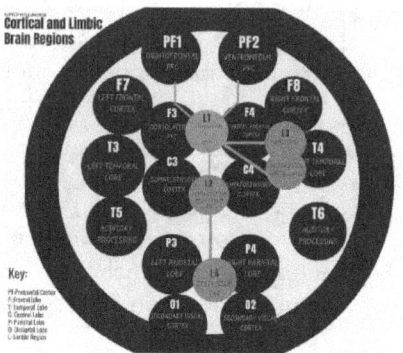

For emotional brain maps, I refer to the location of limbic system structures as limbic regions L1, L2, L3 and L4.

Brain Maps	Brain Region	Functions
	L1	**Limbic Region #1 = L1 Regulation of the Body, Senses, Emotions and Social Ability** The limbic region includes the interfacing middle prefrontal structures, the medial (middle), ventral (front/belly) and orbitofrontal (behind the eyes) portions of the prefrontal cortex and the anterior cingulate cortex (ACC). If our limbic circuits are not strongly integrated with the middle prefrontal region, we may be vulnerable to negative thoughts, mood swings and body symptoms. Regulation of the body and of emotions improves with middle prefrontal integration. The middle prefrontal regions are integral to social and emotional regulation. I call this area the Paleo-Neo Bridge, i.e., the main area of neurodevelopment that we need to focus on to evolve from the paleomammalian brain (the emotional-limbic brain) to our newest brain – the neocortex, aka the social brain. The thalamus is also represented in this region. The thalamus is the

		main pathway of nearly all sensory input to corresponding cortical areas of the brain.
	L2	**Limbic Region #2 = L2** **Cognitive, Motor and Emotional Regulation** This area represents the posterior cingulate cortex (PCC) and the corpus striata complex. The PCC is a major node in the default mode network, which has to do with emotional salience, self-representation and episodic memory retrieval. The corpus striata complex, i.e., the striated nuclei, globus pallidus, nucleus accumbens, entopeduncular nucleus, ventral tegmental area and substantia nigra that are all considered part of a system that manages movement. This system is where cognitive and emotional information converge before coherent behavior follows. Highly evolved brain regions still utilize this system as a final output pathway for behavior. "It seems likely that basal ganglia [corpus striata] circuitry elaborates a primitive feeling of motor presence, which may represent a "primal source of willpower" (Panksepp, 2017).
	L3	**Limbic Region #3 = L3** **Regulation of Unconscious Fear Memories** This area has to do with the amygdala, hippocampus and hypothalamus. The amygdala is the key brain structure used to trigger fear or anxiety in response to threatening stimuli. Unconscious emotional memories in the amygdala are the seat of anxiety disorders. PF1 and PF2 (the higher prefrontal regions, including the orbitofrontal cortex (OFC) and medial prefrontal cortex (mPFC)), send dense inhibitory projections to the lower limbic regions, including the amygdala and hippocampus, in order to modulate the neural activity of fear and anxiety (He, et al., 2014). The hippocampus is involved in the encoding of new memories. It helps us control our emotional response by transforming sensory stimuli into hormonal signals, which then send this information to other parts of the brain that

		control behavior. When we perceive a threat, our hippocampus compares it to previous unconscious dangers. The hippocampus then communicates to our amygdala by sending alerts to the fight-or-flight and hormonal systems. This area also represents the HPA axis. The hypothalamus regulates hormones by sending signals to the pituitary and adrenal glands to maintain homeostasis. When we find ourselves repeatedly responding to internal and external triggers, this self-reinforcing loop may be keeping the hypothalamus and pituitary churning out neurotransmitters and hormones that match our negative emotions and further intensifying the limbic–neural nets, increasing the alarm/stress response.
	L4	**Limbic Region #4 = L4 Cognitive, Sensory-Motor and Emotional Regulation** This region has to do with the cerebellum and the periaqueductal gray area of the midbrain. The posterior lobules of the cerebellum are significantly involved in processes that are associated with cognitive and emotional functions (Depping et al., 2016). In addition to important roles in motor control, it is now thought that the olivo-cerebellar system links to survival networks via the midbrain periaqueductal gray, a structure with a well-known role in expression of survival responses.

Now that we have reviewed general brain areas and functions, let's look at the highly charged neural circuits that exist for each type of overexcitability.

Intellectual Overexcitabilities

Please fill out the following questionnaire to see if this describes you.

Intellectual Overexcitabilities Questionnaire	YES	NO
Very curious and freely approaches new situations	☐	☐
Highly verbal	☐	☐
Analytic thinker	☐	☐
Keen observer	☐	☐
Good at memorizing large amounts of data	☐	☐
Avid reader	☐	☐
Preoccupation with concepts	☐	☐
Detailed planner	☐	☐
Search for truth and understanding	☐	☐
Perseveres in interests	☐	☐
Love of problem solving	☐	☐
Learns new things rapidly	☐	☐
Motivated by ideas	☐	☐
Asks probing questions	☐	☐
Good concentration and ability to maintain intellectual effort	☐	☐

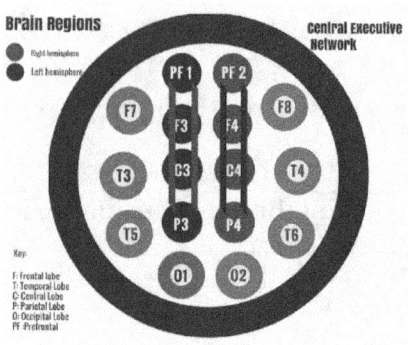

Intellectual Overexcitabilities

Intellectual overexcitabilities (OEs) have to do with a drive towards learning, problem-solving and reflective thinking. According to Dabrowski, those with intellectual OEs love new ideas and have a strong sense of justice. This is demonstrated by a marked need to seek understanding and truth, to gain knowledge and to analyze and synthesize information. Besides high-level creative intelligence, this shows up as rapid information processing and heightened cognitive control.

This brain circuitry is most closely associated with our "executive self," which is our rational decision maker. The executive self is made possible by the Central Executive Network (CEN) which includes two major nodes: the dorsolateral prefrontal cortex (DLPFC) and the posterior parietal cortex (PPC). The CEN is involved in sustained attention, working memory, making decisions and initiating actions.

5 Q Model of Intellectual Overexcitabilities

Translating these concepts into the 5-Q model, we can say that those with intellectual overexcitabilities rely on PF1 and regions of reasoning, data retrieval and working memory (F3, F4, P3, P4).

These regions are used to analyze complex problems and find logical solutions. High activity in F3 area would explain why those with high intelligence are able to handle a lot of concepts and data at one time. F4 has to do with understanding humor, categorizing and defining. This region is also involved with inhibition of responses, maintaining motor coordination, verbal reasoning and problem solving. P3 has to do with rote math and reading, cognitive reasoning, attention, spelling, short-term memory and imagination. P4 is the site related to proprioception that allows us to sense ourselves in space. P4 is also involved in visuomotor control or directing attention as well as maintaining an alert state.

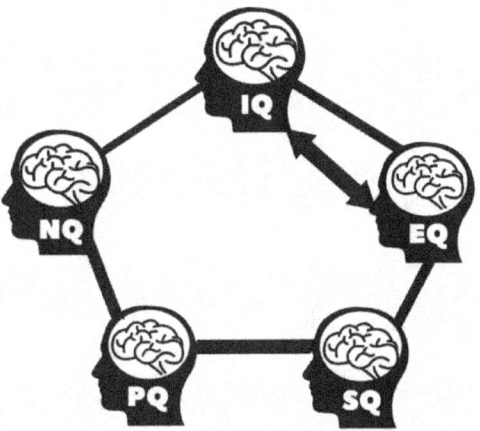

Cognitive Intelligence and Emotional Overexcitabilities

Most people are not aware that people with higher than average intelligence often struggle with emotional regulation, but researchers have found that intellectual and emotional overexcitability are positively correlated (Beduna et al., 2015). Fill out the following questionnaire to see if this describes you.

Emotional Overexcitabilities Questionnaire	YES	NO
Has intense anger or problems controlling anger	☐	☐
Feelings of guilt and sense of responsibility	☐	☐
Inability to handle stress – easily overwhelmed	☐	☐
Identifies with the feelings of others	☐	☐
Has feelings of inadequacy and inferiority	☐	☐
Experiences anxiety	☐	☐
Experiences depression	☐	☐
Painfully sensitive to criticism	☐	☐
Physical response to emotions (stomach aches, headaches)	☐	☐
Struggles with mood swings	☐	☐
Concerned with death	☐	☐
Has strong somatic expressions – blushing, sweaty palms	☐	☐
Has a heightened sense of right and wrong, injustice and hypocrisy	☐	☐

Emotional Overexcitabilities

People with emotional overexcitabilities tend to get overwhelmed by intense emotions and have disproportionate reactions. They might be very self-critical and suffer with feelings of inadequacy, sadness and disappointment. Another characteristic of those with emotional OEs is the tendency to be deeply affected by their feelings and often to respond physically to emotions, e.g., anxiety-induced bowel problems. Being overwhelmed by intense emotions (and not yet knowing how to be in charge of extreme sensitivity and emotional regulation) can be mistaken for anxiety and depression-related disorders. Depression and anxiety are also associated with pro-inflammatory cytokines, which suggests that prolonged stress can influence immunity (Tian et al., 2014).

Learning about our dominant neural nets can help us improve our comfort level in the world. The first thing to recognize is that there may be a lack of top down control from PF1 and PF2 over limbic regions L1, L2, L3 and L4. Also, in the case of emotional overexcitabilities, the hypothalamic-pituitary-adrenal (HPA) axis, the salience network (SN) and the default mode network (DMN) are all likely at play.

It is well known that those who have mood disorders have a hyperactive default mode network (DMN) that stays excitable instead of shutting down. This lends to a highly ruminative cognitive style which is not only associated with increased vulnerability to major depression, but also contributes to symptom severity (Coplan et al., 2012). As with rumination, those who tend to worry more often and more severely score higher on tests of intelligence. Penney et al. (2015) found that verbal intelligence in particular is a positive predictor of worry and rumination, as well as being predictive of severity of both.

All of these states are brought about by heightened neural circuitry in the default mode network (DMN). When we are caught up in self-referencing and worried about the past and future, it keeps this cycle going. This may coactivate the salience network, which in turn may create a hyper focus on what is felt and sensed from the negative thought looping of the DMN.

Further, environmental and psychological threats may prime the HPA to be in a chronic "fight, flight or freeze" response, rendering the nervous system unable to fully relax (Anticevic et al., 2012). In this chronically activated state, the brain stops distinguishing between real and perceived threats and reacts to everything. It's likely that those with emotional overexcitabilities feel perceived stressors/threats more intensely than most people due to chronic evaluation of psychological and environmental stressors, made possible by coactivation of the salience network. This combination in turn may further contribute to anxiety, depression and autoimmune disease.

In this case, we need to learn how to shift out of hyper DMN and/or hyper salience modes and into the central executive network (CEN) or the frontoparietal control network (FPCN) to reframe our worries and change our mood and perspective.

The takeaway is that those with gifted cognitive intelligence, who also have strong emotional reactions, need to honor their intense drives to learn and change the world, especially if it's getting in the way of mental health. Improvements can occur when you train your brain to change states and avoid excessive drives (e.g., to keep ploughing through a project) when you are exhausted. You can start to recognize when you are engaged in intellectual overdrive, for example, and you will immediately be able to start self-regulating with breathing, meditation, music and movement.

EQ - Emotional Intelligence Brain Maps

Now let's discuss the likely brain regions involved in emotional intelligence. Those with high emotional intelligence likely have good connectivity from PF1 and PF2 over the limbic regions. The strength of these regions will yield good top-down control over L1, L2, L3 and L4.

PF1 and PF2 (the higher prefrontal regions, including the orbitofrontal cortex (OFC) and medial prefrontal cortex (mPFC)) send dense inhibitory projections to the lower limbic regions, including L1, L2, L3 and L4. L1 has to do with regulation of the body, senses, emotions and social ability. L2 is related to cognitive, motor and emotional regulation. L3 is related to regulation of unconscious fear memories. L4 has to do with cognitive, sensory-motor and emotional regulation.

Secrets for Improving Emotional Intelligence

1. Include neuroplastic techniques like meditation, yoga, acupuncture, aromatherapy
2. Switch brain networks, e.g., from hyper-DMN and hyper-salience networks to FPCN
3. Anti-inflammatory diet; include Omega-3 EPA/DHA, B Complex and Vitamin D
4. Practice natural ways to increase GABA, serotonin and dopamine, include exercise, clean diet and a combination of dietary supplements, such as Gabatone, Dopatone, Serotone
5. Use music to meet the needs of: safety, relaxation, happiness, satisfaction, belonging
6. Emo-Sensory Therapy

Imaginational Overexcitabilities

Fill out the following questionnaire to see if this describes you.

Imaginational Overexcitabilities Questionnaire	YES	NO
Loves symbolism and metaphors	☐	☐
Has a persistent curiosity	☐	☐
Has a good sense of humor	☐	☐
Engages in animistic and magical thinking	☐	☐
Has a love of poetry, music, drama	☐	☐
Has a facility for invention and fantasy	☐	☐
Has vivid dreams	☐	☐
Has a tendency to mix truth with fiction	☐	☐
Has a facility for detailed visualization and imagination	☐	☐
Uses intuition and hunches	☐	☐
Sees the big picture	☐	☐
Bored by routine	☐	☐
Can connect seemingly unrelated ideas	☐	☐
Has unusual ideas or perceptions	☐	☐
Acutely aware of own and others' feelings	☐	☐

Imaginational Overexcitability

Imaginational overexcitability refers to having elaborate daydreams and fantasies. For the most part, imagination is an amazing asset. The downside of it is that some people end up imagining the worst outcome of any situation, which may make them fearful of new situations. Those with imaginational OEs exhibit enhanced perception, attention and memory, which may make the world too intense and lead to symptoms including withdrawal and social avoidance. They may forego interpersonal contact because of fear of disapproval, criticism or rejection. They may also be preoccupied with being criticized in social situations and tend to view themselves as being socially inept or inferior to others.

Giftedness can involve an affective awareness, which lends to a high perceptivity of the environment. Affective awareness comes from emotional responses to sensory experiences and the meaning created in response to perceptions. The bottom line is that neurons in the brain may be especially sensitive and flexible in those who have intense perception, hyper-focus, strong memory and strong emotions. This increased engagement of neural networks may allow some people to learn more quickly but may also result in stronger fear responses and stronger fear memories. When imagination is relentless and negative, some may suffer from diseases of rumination including anxiety and depression, which we now know may drive autoimmune reactions in a vicious cycle. So, if you have that kind of sensitivity, you really are best served by honoring it, respecting it and being determined to choose situations and people that nourish you and avoid those that drain you.

Imaginational Overexcitabilities Brain Regions (PF2, L2)

Translating this into dominant neural networks, those with imaginational overexcitabilities may be prone to getting stuck in the default mode network (DMN). In this case, they largely rely on PF2 and L2. The default mode network is thought to be the neurological basis for the self. That is, the ego - or the autobiographical self - is generated by the functions of the DMN.

Remember that the default mode network is active when our mind is wandering e.g., when we are thinking about ourself and others, remembering the past or imagining the future. L2 represents the location of the posterior cingulate cortex (PCC), which is a major node involved in the default mode network (DMN) that has to do with self-representation. PF2 is the area that is active when we self-reflect and use self-control. If we are caught in incessant self-reflection, we may not be as efficient with self-control.

On a neurobiological level, excessive functioning of the DMN creates hyper-plasticity and hyper-functionality. This not only alters your perceptions and cognitive functions but also (especially if incessant and negative) may engage the HPA and the amygdala as well as the salience network (SN).

The link between our attention to and perception of everyday life experience is made possible via the salience network (SN). Both the insula and the anterior cingulate cortex (key nodes of the network) analyze information from all over the brain to work out what is the most salient. This process relies on the limbic region and is involved in our sense of intuition. However, when the salience and default mode networks over-communicate with each other and with other networks, our representation of our self may become either more fluid or more chaotic. On the one hand, this can allow more novel problem-solving pathways to be opened up, leading to enhanced insight and intuition. On the other hand, the salience network may increase the significance of usually unimportant or negative things.

The key point is that those with imaginational overexcitabilities need to cherish their creative minds without getting too caught up in imaginary worlds. Having the support and encouragement of a few good friends and/or a good therapist, plus some solid neuroplastic practices, can be very helpful. We need to make the leap from the trappings of our imaginational overexcitabilities to more mature and accurate intuitive intelligence.

NQ - Intuitive Intelligence Brain Activity (PF1, PF2)

Translating this into neural networks, intuitive intelligence refers to top-down control from the prefrontal regions over the limbic regions. If we are stuck in ruminative neural networks, there may be less activity in other regions of the brain that aid in logic, intuition and metacognition, namely, the prefrontal regions required for intuitive intelligence. Essentially, we can shift brain networks from a hyper DMN and/or salience network, to the central executive network (which is related to logic) or the frontoparietal control network (FPCN), which has to do with metacognition, reappraisal and response inhibition.

Prefrontal Regions 1 and 2

PF1 is the judge area of the brain. It's the part of the brain that filters negative inputs, decides, notices errors and provides reasons. PF2 is the area that is active when we ponder our sense of self, use self-control and restrain our impulses. If our imagination runs wild, we can rely on higher brain function to alert us to any inaccuracies in interpreting our circumstances and getting stuck in imagining the worst. Supporting the prefrontal region will yield better top down control over limbic regions L1-L4. L1 has to do with regulation of the body, senses, emotions and social ability. L2 is related to cognitive, motor and emotional regulation. L3 is related to regulation of unconscious fear memories. L4 has to do with cognitive, sensory-motor and emotional regulation. See the "optimizing self-regulation skills" section below for ways to support the prefrontal region.

Sensual Overexcitabilities

Please fill out the following questionnaire to see if this describes you.

Sensual Overexcitabilities Questionnaire	YES	NO
Very perceptive and insightful	☐	☐
Delights in nature, beautiful objects, form and color	☐	☐
Delights in music and the sound of words	☐	☐
Has enhanced sensory and aesthetic pleasure	☐	☐
Highly intuitive to others' feelings	☐	☐
Thin-skinned or feels emotionally porous	☐	☐
Startles easily	☐	☐
Sensitive to perfumes, foods, alcohol, etc.	☐	☐
Thrives in an encouraging environment	☐	☐
Avoids negative and/or violent movies	☐	☐
Experiences sensory overload	☐	☐
Easily overwhelmed at parties or large crowds	☐	☐
Easily bothered by noise, lights and smells	☐	☐
Dislikes words and events that hurt animals or people	☐	☐
Requires a large amount of downtime or alone time	☐	☐

Sensual Overexcitabilities

Many people with anxiety, depression, sensory processing, learning disorders and autoimmune disease share the same trait of extreme sensitivity – whether it be environmental, emotional or physical. It's a sense of needing to protect the self that is reflected in our psychology (and behavior), but the backdrop has never been explicated in a way that fits a neurobiological understanding. In the 5Q model, sensual overexcitabilities may be related to the entire sensory processing spectrum. The dominant networks and structures include the hypothalamic-pituitary-adrenal (HPA) axis, the salience network (SN), as well as the somatosensory cortex and the thalamus. In those that have high sensitivity (HSPs) and sensory overresponsivity (SOR), the thalamus, HPA and salience network (SN) are likely the primary areas to focus on. Those with sensory processing disorder should also support the somatosensory cortex and especially the temporal, occipital and parietal lobes.

Sensual Overexcitability – Brain Areas C3, C4, F7, F8, P3, P4, T3, T4, T5, T6, O1, O2, L1-L4.

Having sensual overexcitabilities means that your dominant neural nets are likely within the somatosensory cortex, the frontal cortex, the thalamus, and the parietal, occipital and temporal lobes. The somatosensory cortex integrates sensory information (interoception) and spatial awareness (proprioception). The frontal cortex (specifically the insula) has to do with integrating cognitive, sensory and emotional information. The thalamus is the main pathway of nearly all sensory input to corresponding cortical areas of the brain. The parietal lobes are responsible for processing sensory information from the body and from the environment. Functional connectivity between the parietal and frontal lobes also yields non-verbal physical information of where you are in space/time and how you are relating to others.

The temporal lobes process language, verbal, and emotional non-verbal memory. Just because the neural nets are dominant, it does not mean they are functionally connected. Gaining an understanding of the regions and neural nets involved will help you create a treatment plan for functional integration. The following regions likely play a role in creating sensory processing issues.

Central Regions 3 and 4

C3/C4 is located on the top of the primary somatosensory cortex. This part of your brain is responsible for processing touch, interoception and proprioception.

Frontal Regions 7 and 8

F7 is part of the frontal cortex, which integrates sensory, cognitive and emotional information. This area relates to the sensitivities that you notice. F8 is recruited for emotional regulation, social inhibition and emotional/personal values.

Parietal Regions 3 and 4

P3 is part of the mirror neuron system and is involved in copying emotional tones, innuendo and non-verbal memory. P4 is the site related to proprioception that allows us to sense ourselves in space. P4 is also involved in visuomotor control or directing attention, as well as maintaining an alert state.

Temporal Regions 3 and 4

T3 handles language, including verbal memory, phonological processing, diction, grammar and voice tone. T3 has to do with hearing words of self/others while T4 has to do with discerning tone of voice and weighing the motivation and intent of others. When humming, speaking and listening to music, T3 and T4 are recruited.

Temporal Regions 5 and 6

T5 is recruited when we are curious about what someone is thinking and when we receive social feedback. T6 is used when we are making predictions, thinking symbolically and strategizing about the future. T6 also lends to emotional understanding, facial recognition and auditory processing. T5 and T6 are both involved in social feedback.

Occipital Regions O1 and O2

O1 is where we mentally visualize and scan the environment for lost items. O2 has to do with abstract visualization and visual impressions.

Limbic Regions 1, 2, 3 and 4

L1 has to do with regulation of the body, senses, emotions and social ability. L2 is related to cognitive, motor and emotional regulation. L3 is related to regulation of unconscious fear memories. L4 has to do with cognitive, sensory-motor and emotional regulation.

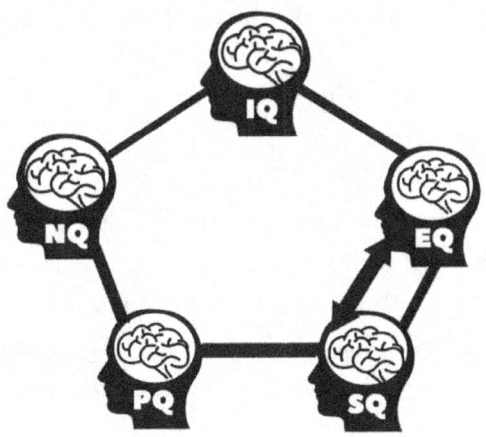

Sensual Overexcitabillity Affects Emotional Regulation

Sensitive people are generally more self-other reflective and much more aware of subtleties in the environment. They may have trouble setting personal boundaries and separating their own feelings and needs from those of others. As a result, they tend to absorb the emotions of people around them.

While highly sensitive people are generally more emotionally aware, emotional reactivity and regulation may be an issue. The downside is that this internalized processing loop, which is going on in the background along with the tendency to absorb the emotions of others, is the energy zapper that they need to know about.

Those with sensual overexcitabilities may tend to be empathic and prone to high stress due to high levels of their own and others' emotions. These personality tendencies make them prone to developing an unhealthy stress response, which we now know fuels anxiety, depression, unintegrated sensory processing and autoimmune reactions. Susceptibility to stress, plus the tendency to neglect one's own needs while putting others first, can make people emote and behave in ways that feel incongruent with what they really feel internally. The problem is that people in this situation haven't identified the pattern and the world is just fine accepting their agreeableness.

If we are consumed and over-powered by sensory input or lacking the correct kind of input, this can also create emotional intensity. Once we wake up to the nature of the brain circuitry behind our hypersensitivity and/or sensory processing challenges, we can begin to employ neuroplastic techniques to improve functional connectivity in all areas of the brain related to sensory integration.

The Sensory Processing Spectrum

While it is well known that people with ADD, ADHD and autism suffer with Sensory Processing Disorders, there are many more people who suffer from Sensory Processing Sensitivities. In her book, *The Highly Sensitive Person*, Dr. Elaine Aron explores the neuroscience and psychological research behind Sensory Processing Sensitivity (SPS) and Environmental Sensitivity. SPS is considered a trait that has evolved in twenty percent of the human population as a survival strategy. Although not considered a disorder, the problem is that people with high SPS can suffer from overstimulation and may go to great lengths to protect themselves (Aron, 1996).

Sensory Processing (Integration) Disorder (SPD) on the other hand, is considered a neurological disorder that involves the senses: the vestibular system, interoception, proprioception, motor control, balance and spatial awareness. In SPD, sensory information is not properly integrated in the brain, which may result in altered responses to external stimuli, causing overstimulation. So, while overstimulation is involved in both cases, the underlying cause is different.

Again, while Sensory Processing Sensitivity is not considered a disorder, many of the symptoms overlap with Sensory Processing Disorder. Overlapping symptoms of SPD and SPS include hypersensitivity to sound, sight and touch, general overload of stimulation and an inability to regulate emotions.

Researchers have found that adults who are sensory overresponsive (SOR), have much higher levels of anxiety and depression (compared to healthy adults) and that this was also correlated with a perceived absence of social support (Kinnealey, 2011). Separately, adults with mental health issues also show signs of sensory processing difficulties when trying to negotiate the demands of everyday life (Brown et al., 2006). Further, Sensory Processing Sensitivities can also affect sleep quality in healthy individuals who are hypersensitive to tactile, auditory and visual stimuli (Engel-Yeger, 2012).

The goal for all is to help integrate stimuli into experience. Learning about genetic traits like Sensory Processing Sensitivity can help us create a supportive environment. Neuroplastic techniques like meditation, music, sound meditations, walks in nature, yoga, emo-sensory therapy and essential oils can be added to improve overall brain connectivity. This approach's aim is to increase neruo-immuo-plasticity via preferable emotional and sensory pathways, leading to increased tolerance of sensitivities. This creates a greater ability to process the input from the world around us.

When we view emotional and sensory deficits as a right brain deficiency, we can identify brain areas that need support, e.g., the prefrontal cortex, the temporal, occipital and parietal lobes, the somatosensory and motor cortices, the right insular cortex (for sensing oneself internally), the basal ganglia (for sensing one's body in relation to the environment) and/or the cerebellum, which has to do with timing and rhythm.

Sensory Processing Sensitivity and HSPs
Many people with autoimmune, learning and affective disorders have a highly sensitive sensory system. They may be sensitive to noise, smells, loud sounds and tend to skip exhausting social events. Sensory processing sensitivity (SPS) is considered a trait in which a person experiences greater sensitivity to external stimuli and higher emotional reactivity than the rest of the world. Those who have this trait are described as HSPs (highly sensitive people).

Highly sensitive people are known to be overstimulated easily, find noise distracting and chaotic situations disorienting. They are the empaths who are finely attuned to feeling everything that others are feeling. They also need a lot of personal space and downtime to process all of the sensory data that they take in.

Extreme responsiveness to stressful stimuli and social situations may make HSPs prone to anxiety. In fact, brain imaging showed that this reactivity reflects a hyperresponsive amygdala, the area of the brain that governs the fear response (Kagan et al., 2004). A hyperresponsive amygdala can lead to hypervigilance - being on the constant lookout for danger. This hypersensitivity can also create undesirable immune reactions, including allergies and autoimmunity.

A lesser-known fact about those with sensory processing issues is that the degree to which they respond to sensory and/or emotional and social stimuli may be a clue that the brain's timing is off in one or more brain regions. When we consider how sensitivity is occurring in the brain, we can imagine that this ability comes from recruiting specific areas of the brain repeatedly. The main areas involved in sensory processing and integration include the mirror neuron system, the anterior insular cortex, the anterior cingulate cortex, the thalamus, the somatosensory cortex, the frontal, occipital, parietal and temporal lobes. Let's consider the importance of the mirror neuron system as well as the anterior insular cortex in sensory and emotional processing.

Mirror Neurons

Functional Magnetic Resonance Imaging (fMRI) of HSPs reveals that brains of individuals who are highly sensitive respond more powerfully to emotional images than individuals who are not highly sensitive (Acevedo et al., 2014). From a neurobiological standpoint, higher levels of awareness and emotional responsiveness in highly sensitive people correlate with greater activity in the mirror neuron system and the anterior insular cortex areas of the brain.

A special network of brain cells, called mirror neurons, subconsciously communicates our emotional response to what we see and hear, and orchestrates our emotional and social development. Mirror neurons drive the non-verbal communication system, e.g., when we see facial expressions and body postures in others, our mirror neurons trigger the same internal responses and we make instinctive movements to mirror the posture and emotion of what we see.

This mirroring is a normal part of social bonding. When we see others smile and we smile back, it means our mirror neurons are working well. If we find that we're not very adept at nonverbal communication, our mirror neurons are likely not firing well. This may lead us to struggle with distinguishing others' emotions and intentions. On the other hand, having an increase of activity in the mirror neuron system may also make us more sensitive to others' emotions.

The Anterior Insular Cortex

The anterior insular cortex is a key node of the salience network (SN), which is recruited for cognitive, sensory and emotional integration. Even though it's not technically part of the limbic region, the insula acts as a relay station for communication between body (via the spinal cord and brainstem), limbic region and cortex. The anterior insular cortex is involved in interoception, emotional regulation and empathy. The insula is also involved in sudden insight, consciousness and sense of selfhood. Working with the middle prefrontal regions (ACC, vmPFC and orbitofrontal cortex (OFC)), the insula is thought to serve as a conduit for the flow of information that allows us to form pictures of the state of our own bodies and of one another's minds. This is referred to as theory of mind (ToM). Deficits in this function are referred to as *mind-blindness.*

Knowing more about the brain regions involved in levels of sensitivity, gives us insight into how this comes about from a brain-based level.

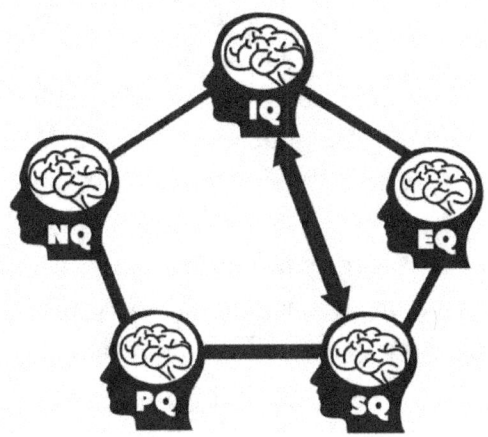

Cognitive Intelligence and Sensory Processing Challenges

The overlap between sensory processing challenges and intellectual giftedness may include a heightened awareness of sensory input, having a reactive limbic system (poor self-regulation and emotions), trouble with change and transitions, difficulty with social interactions, preference to being alone, lack of social graces and reading of social cues, along with rigid and narrow interests (Voss, 2017). These symptoms may be due to high synchrony (or hyper-connectivity) of cortices and resultant increase in entropy. They also may be due to hypoconnectivity of the prefrontal cortex to sensory and emotional regulation areas of the brain.

Autism Spectrum Disorder

While ASD is now considered a complex neuro-immune and inflammatory disorder, Dr. Leo Kanner was the first to propose the link between gifted intelligence and autism in 1943. He described children who were highly intelligent and able to remember and reproduce complex patterns but who also displayed "a powerful desire for aloneness" and "an obsessive insistence on persistent sameness" (Kanner, 1943). Hans Asperger later described highly intelligent boys, who had specific obsessive interests and trouble with social interactions, as another form of autism that became known as Asperger's syndrome (Asperger, 1944, Frith, 1991).

Currently there is evidence that corroborates early observations of gifted intelligence, suggesting that enhanced neural circuitry may be behind high functioning ASD. The brain areas thought to be involved with superior functioning include logical-working memory, verbal fluency and vocabulary (Clark et al., 2016).

However, in some cases of ASD, portions of the frontal lobes may not be independent enough to coordinate and integrate brain functions, e.g., attending, planning, arranging, inhibiting, delaying and restraining our emotional reactions. In some cases it has been found that the parietal lobes are frequently not organizing and processing sensory information from the body and from the environment well enough. There may also be increased white matter in the frontal lobes, the cerebellum and other areas related to higher order processing. In addition, there may also be aberrant connectivity (hyper or hypo) from the temporal, occipital and parietal lobes to the prefrontal cortex. This may translate as a diminished ability to process sensory-motor (including proprioception, interoception), cognitive and emotional stimuli.

Functional connectivity between the parietal and frontal lobes also yields non-verbal physical information regarding where you are in space/time and how you are relating to others. It turns out that this is important information in order for people to be socially successful. Not surprisingly, feeling physically disconnected is also related to social and emotional immaturity. If you do not feel safe and grounded, you may not able to form normal emotional relationships with family members and friends. If you lack this self-perception, this can lead to poor social skills. When you don't feel or sense your body well, it may also be hard for you to accurately read your own emotions and therefore those of others.

The salience network (SN) has also been consistently found to be atypical in autism spectrum disorders (ASD) (Green et al., 2016). Altered SN connectivity can lead to altered brain activity during information processing, which can lead to sensory overresponsivity (SOR), not only in ASD but also in other disorders related to difficulty downregulating brain responses to sensory stimuli. In addition, basic sensory information becomes overly salient to individuals with SOR, leading to hyperfocusing of attention on sensory information.

Interestingly, Velázquez et al (2013) found that the brains of autistic children produce 42% more information when in a resting state than non-autistic children, suggesting increased excitatory connections. This finding, along with findings from studies on autistic animals, led researchers Kamila and Henry Markram to develop the Intense World Theory (IWT) of autism spectrum disorder, which proposes hyper-functioning of local neural microcircuits, characterized by hyper-reactivity and hyper-plasticity in emotional and sensory circuits (Markram and Markram, 2010). The IWT characterizes those with autism as intellectually gifted individuals who see and feel so intensely that they "must engage in avoidance and lock down behaviors in order to for them to escape" (Karpinski et al., 2017).

Since the right hemisphere of the brain regulates sensory and emotional integration, non-verbal learning, attention and socially appropriate behavior, those with decreased right brain activity may have trouble reading body language, maintaining eye contact, and regulating sensory overload, mood and repetitive behaviors.

The good news is that you can make improvements in functional connectivity with customized activities. Supporting functional connectivity in distinct regions of the brain (frontal and prefrontal lobes, somatosensory cortex, thalamus, temporal, parietal and occipital lobes) may prove to have great results in reducing outward indications of ASD. See "secrets for improving sensory intelligence" below for a short list of things to try.

Sensory Processing Disorder
Sensory processing disorders (sometimes termed sensory integration disorders) can affect one or more of our senses. One person may feel dizzy in response to visually challenging designs, another may be very sensitive to loud sound, while someone else may not be efficiently processing (proprioceptive) messages from the muscles and joints, which can show up as poor motor skills. SPD is typically found in those with autism, learning disabilities, developmental coordination disorder or other diagnoses.

Children affected with SPD have been shown to have less white matter microstructure in the brain areas that involve sensory processing and integration, which may help explain some of the challenges children with SPD have (Owen et al., 2013). Decreased white matter microstructure is considered the biological basis for SPD that sets it apart from other sensory processing conditions.

Remember that white matter forms the connectome that links different brain regions and is considered essential for perceiving, thinking and action. White matter circuitry affects cognitive processing, auditory integration, social skills, memory and attention. In SPD, the dysfunction may specifically have to do with reduced white matter connectivity in between the parietal and occipital lobes (which play a large part in sensory processing and integration), along with reduced connectivity in the temporal lobes.

A lesser-known fact is that the temporal lobe is an area of the brain that not only receives input from the senses (especially hearing), but also contributes to social-emotional processing. Quiescent temporal lobes can lead to social and emotional regulation issues. Some have referred to kids with SPD as "out of sync" children. Their use of language is normal yet they may have trouble with just about everything else - especially emotional regulation and distraction. They are less able to process information efficiently and sometimes get left out.

A remedy could be to improve the functional connectivity in the temporal lobes as well as in the parietal and occipital lobes for better sensory perception, processing and integration. Acupuncture may be the most helpful therapy for this, as it can be performed directly on the scalp to improve the connectivity of these lobes.

Perception of Sensory Information

Our perception of life and the environment relies on our senses to create the world that we see. However, it is important to understand that our perceptions are modified by the neural resources available to us and can sometimes be wrong. Ultimately, perception depends on functional connectivity in all of the lobes of the brain, especially the occipital lobe (vision), somatosensory cortex (sensation) and temporal lobe (sounds). In essence, your perceptions are only as good as your sensory system.

Sensory Integration
The goal of treatment should be to help build functional neural pathways that can lead to efficient responses to information flowing into the brain through the senses. This is admittedly time-consuming and requires frequent repetition but it is necessary. Specifically, supporting functional connectivity (of the prefrontal and frontal lobes, somatosensory cortex, thalamus, temporal, parietal and occipital lobes), with the use of sensory strategies, will support emotions, learning and behavior not only in those with sensory processing issues but also in the aging adult population.

SQ - Sensory Intelligence
A healthy sensory system is essential to healthy brain function because it is the sole driver of stimulation to the brain. Besides the sensory processing spectrum that we just covered, sensory processing deficits can also result from neurodegeneration in aging adults. In many cases, sensitivity to noise, challenges with attention and difficulties with emotional regulation can result. Not surprisingly, the treatment is the same. The focus is on improving functional connectivity in the regions that need it most. Essentially, it comes down to emotional and sensory integration (aka vertical integration) and getting good at regulating the flow of information from the right to the left-brain (aka horizontal integration).

When we work at the level of cause in brain-based imbalances, we may see our undesirable tendencies, patterns and symptoms resolve themselves. For example, if we tend to experience anxiety and we practice one or several sensory strategies daily for six weeks, we can lock in neuroplastic changes that may result in feeling calmer and more balanced with greater mental clarity. This boosts our confidence and makes for positive learning. See below for more examples of brain-based therapies to include.

Brain Areas Involved in Sensory Intelligence

To promote sensory intelligence, we can look at the sensory integration areas of the brain and other specific regions that need regulating - for example, the somatosensory cortex and/or regions for spatial (parietal lobe) or auditory (temporal lobe) processing. We can also learn to reign in our highly engaged emotional brain when (through unconscious connections with others) we get ensnared in negative dynamics that overstimulate and overwhelm our sensitive neurology.

Sensory intelligence may be improved with neuroplastic techniques. When you investigate the areas of the brain that are involved, you will start to gain insight about the need to improve functional connectivity among these brain regions to integrate cognitive, emotional and sensory inputs. The more information you have, the more you can find appropriate strategies to keep heightened reactions from limiting your life. Focus on all lobes, cortices and regions that improve sensory integration: PF1, PF2, C3, C4, F7, F8, P3, P4, T3, T4, T5, T6, O1, O2, L1, L2, L3, L4.

Prefrontal Regions

PF1 and PF2 (the higher prefrontal regions, including the orbitofrontal cortex (OFC) and medial prefrontal cortex (mPFC)) send dense inhibitory projections to the lower limbic regions, including the amygdala and hippocampus, in order to modulate the neural activity of fear and anxiety, which may be triggered by sensory overload.

Frontal Regions F7, F8
F7 is a part of the frontal cortex that integrates sensory and emotional information. F8 is related to social inhibition and is also used for emotional regulation.

Parietal Lobes P3, P4
P3 is part of the mirror neuron system and is involved in copying emotional tones, innuendo, nuance and non-verbal memory. It also has to do with identifying objects, symbol recognition, rote math, reading, spelling, cognitive reasoning, attention, short-term memory and imagination. P4 is the site related to proprioception that allows us to sense ourselves in space. P4 is also involved in visuomotor control, or directing attention, as well as maintaining an alert state.

Central Regions C3 and C4
C3 and C4 house the somatosensory cortex, which integrates sensory information (e.g., interoception, touch, pressure, temperature, pain and spatial awareness (proprioception)).

Occipital Regions O1 and O2
O1 is where we mentally visualize and scan the environment for lost items. O2 has to do with abstract visualization and visual impressions.

Temporal Regions (T3, T4, T5 and T6)
These regions handle language, including diction, grammar, voice tone, verbal memory and phonological processing.

Limbic Regions 1, 2, 3 and 4
L1 has to do with regulation of the body, senses, emotions and social ability. L2 is related to cognitive, motor and emotional

regulation. L3 is related to regulation of unconscious fear memories. L4 has to do with cognitive, sensory-motor and emotional regulation.

Improving Sensory Skills
Since so many people with right hemisphere imbalances struggle with sensory processing issues, it is important to have tools to remedy sensory processing areas that need it most. For sensory deficits in smell, touch, vision, hearing and/or balance, you can start by improving every processing function that is low, so it can sync up with the rest of the brain.

Choose activities to improve areas that need it most, e.g., proprioception, touch, visual, auditory and olfactory processing. In any sensory integration approach, the key is to focus on intensity and repetition. Aim for daily or at least one hour/day, three times each week, of intense activities and stimulation, along with good nutrition and behavior strategies. Add these to basic activities like physical exercise to stimulate overall brain growth and development.

Simultaneously growing the frontal cortex through physical and cognitive stimulation will also improve control over the (impulsive-emotional) limbic brain and brainstem activity. Finally, any intervention that addresses sensory processing difficulties needs to include strategies for decreasing the sympathetic response (fight or flight) and increasing vagal tone and the parasympathetic (rest and digest) response with the use of relaxation techniques. Here are some sensory strategies and tools to help self-regulate throughout the day.

Secrets for Improving Sensory Intelligence – The Short List
1. Hearing - sound meditation and music
2. Smell - olfactory stimulation with essential oils
3. Touch - massage therapy
4. Body socks
5. Restorative yoga and pranayama
6. <u>Anti-inflammatory diet</u>, including Omega-3 EPA/DHA, B Complex and Vitamin D
7. Include natural ways to increase serotonin and GABA with exercise, adequate protein and a combination of dietary supplements, such as Serotone and Gabatone
8. Use music to meet the needs of safety, relaxation, happiness, satisfaction and belonging
9. <u>Emo-Sensory Therapy</u>

Please see the "brain-based therapies" section below for more sensory-motor exercises that may apply.

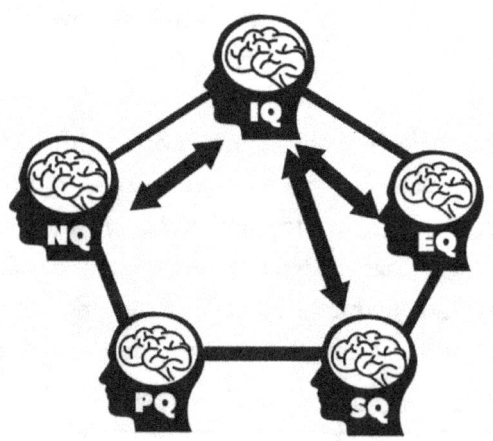

Intellectual Overexcitabilities and Physiological Responses
Those with gifted cognitive intelligence have enhanced functional connectivity in the dorsolateral prefrontal cortex (DLPFC) and

the posterior parietal cortex (PPC), i.e., the two major nodes of the Central Executive Network (CEN). Due to this increased connectivity, those with an overexcitable cognitive ability tend toward hyper-reactivity of the central nervous system which, in turn, can lead to various physiological consequences, including asthma, sensory processing sensitivity and autoimmune disease (Chang et al., 2013).

In the 5Q model, this may be due to a combination of intellectual plus imaginational, sensual and emotional overexcitabilities that need regulation. Dabrowski's characterization of imaginational, emotional, sensual and intellectual overexcitabilities are a good entry point into understanding these states. As we can see, each of these overexcitabilities relate to the three main brain networks involved in physiological responses: the default mode network (DMN), the salience network (SN) and central executive networks (CEN). In my model, we can consider physiological responses as stemming from over engagement in the three main brain networks: the salience network, DMN and the CEN along with coactivation of the HPA. Once we understand more about the networks involved, we can work with them.

HYPER-BRAIN HYPER-BODY

HYPER-SALIENCE HYPER-FOCUS AND HYPER-RUMINATION

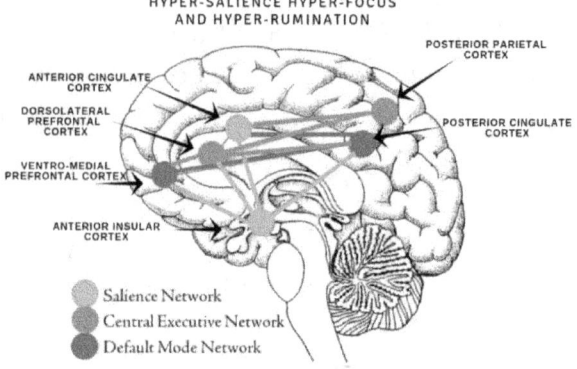

The DMN, the SN and the CEN typically don't get activated at the same time, but it seems as if people with heightened cognitive ability and physiological responses are "wired" differently, causing brain systems that don't typically work together to get over engaged with each other and create too much entropy in the brain. What I am positing is that it is this increase in entropy that makes the brain both more creative *and* vulnerable to "blow outs" or flares. Then, the right hemisphere, with decreased emotional, sensory and cognitive control, manifests as hyper-body responses.

Normal functioning of the networks shows that they interact in relatively fixed ways. For example, the central executive network (CEN) and the default mode network (DMN) are anti-correlated, tending to have more control at different times depending on what task is at hand. The salience network decides what is most important to attend to and switches between the DMN and the CEN. The salience network (SN) discovers errors and failed predictions and engages the other networks so that they can learn from this mistake.

However, the effect of over engagement between networks might help to explain how different levels of overexcitabilities might come about. Heightened neural circuitry in all three brain networks, along with coactivation of the HPA, may render less top down influence from the prefrontal regions over the rest of the brain and result in sensual, imaginational and emotional excitabilities and, inevitably, autoimmune disease and other physiological responses.

At the end of the day, the fallout from over engagement of these highly charged networks is that it can create hyper-reactivity and hyper-plasticity, which may lead to cognitive consequences of hyper-perception, hyper-attention, hyper-memory and hyper-emotionality. We need to know that our symptoms can be driven by overly strong reactions to experiences that train the brain into hyper-preferences, which may further be accelerated by emotionally charged experiences and trauma. This perfect storm of brain activity may lead to obsessively detailed information processing, a painfully intense experience of the world, and resultant physiological responses. Knowing how to work with each of our highly charged neural nets is imperative for anyone suffering at the effect of their overexcitabilities.

Psychomotor Overexcitabilities

Please fill out the following questionnaire to see if this describes you.

Psychomotor Overexcitabilities Questionnaire	YES	NO
Rapid speech	☐	☐
Likes competition - thrives on challenges	☐	☐
Has issues with sleeplessness	☐	☐
Compulsive organizing	☐	☐
Fidgety – can't sit still	☐	☐
Feels out of step with others	☐	☐
Prefers fast action and sports	☐	☐
Has nervous habits and tics	☐	☐
Workaholic	☐	☐
Marked excitation and acting out	☐	☐
Poor impulse control	☐	☐
Prefers intense physical activity	☐	☐
Hyperactive	☐	☐
Impatient and easily frustrated	☐	☐
Poor coordination	☐	☐

Psychomotor Overexcitability

Psychomotor overexcitability refers to heightened neuromuscular activity. This can be expressed as high energy, rapid speech and a need for constant motion. This restlessness makes it difficult to sit still and concentrate and may include acting impulsively or compulsively. Those with psychomotor OEs can also be extremely competitive and may also like to engage in adrenaline-stimulating activities. Symptoms may look like obsessive-compulsive disorder (OCD) or be mistaken for attention deficit hyperactivity disorder (ADHD). Brain areas involved include regions F3, F4, F7, F8, P3, P4, C3, C4 as well as limbic regions L1, L2, L3, L4, without much top down control from the prefrontal cortex.

Frontal Regions F3, F4, F7, F8

F3 is considered the seat of planning, sustained attention and working memory. F4 is involved with inhibition of responses, maintaining motor coordination, verbal reasoning and problem solving. F7 is a part of the frontal cortex that integrates cognitive, sensory and emotional information. F8 is also required for emotional regulation.

Parietal Lobes P3, P4

P3 has to do with identifying objects, symbol recognition, rote math, reading, spelling, cognitive reasoning, attention, short-term memory and imagination. P4 is the site that allows us to sense ourselves in space (proprioception). Those with psychomotor OEs who don't have a good sense of themselves in space may be clumsy and tend to bump into things.

Central Regions C3 and C4

C3 and C4 house the somatosensory cortex, which integrates sensory information (interoception) and spatial awareness (proprioception).

Limbic Regions 1, 2, 3 and 4

L1 has to do with regulation of the body, senses, emotions and social ability. L2 is related to cognitive, motor and emotional regulation. L3 is related to regulation of unconscious fear memories. L4 has to do with cognitive, sensory-motor and emotional regulation.

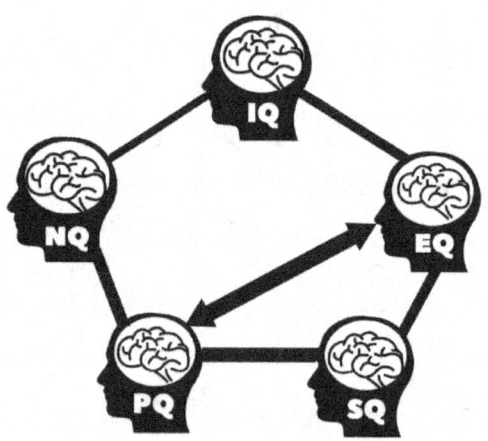

Psychomotor Overexcitabilities Affect Emotional Regulation

People with psychomotor overexcitabilities may not have a good sense of their bodies and may have poor muscle tone or trouble with balance and coordination. Interestingly, when looked at as a lack of timing and coordination, this can also show up as poor social skills where people may say inappropriate things and have a hard time making friends.

Consider for example that hyperactive and sensation-seeking behavior is their brain's way of trying to ground themselves in their experience. Yet, you can easily see that there is a lack of smooth psychomotor activity. If they also have a poor sense of their body in space, this can lead to self-doubt and frustration, which may result in feeling anxious, depressed and socially awkward. If we can train ourselves to understand the ways we communicate through our behavior, we can explore how this actually impacts our emotions and also our social abilities.

From a neurobiological standpoint, this process is rooted in a hyperfunctional motor cortex and a lack of functional connectivity (and therefore lack of top down control) from the prefrontal cortex to the limbic-emotional brain. When the prefrontal cortex isn't functioning up to par, the intention setting mode of the brain is unreliable and in need of support. In a sense, ADHD (as well as self and emotional regulation issues) can be characterized as an intention deficit disorder. That is, the prefrontal cortex isn't mature enough to set intentions and regulate emotions.

From a functional neurology point of view, the right hemisphere relates to emotional and sensory-motor integration. If the right hemisphere is deficient, it can result in impulsivity and even aggressive and socially inappropriate behavior. The remedy is to improve vertical integration of body sensations and emotions on the right side along with supporting the flow of information from the right hemisphere to the left (aka horizontal integration). This will lead to hemispheric balance.

Tailoring sensory-motor and other activities that improve functional connectivity can lead to a reduction of emotional and behavioral symptoms. Essentially, we are trying to move toward developing the dorsal attention network (DAN) for sustained attention, the central executive network (CEN) to improve working memory, the frontoparietal control network (FPCN) for metacognition, reappraisal and intention setting and the striato-pallido-thalamo-cortical-network (SPTCN) for extinction learning.

PQ - Secrets to Improving Psychomotor Intelligence

Ways to decrease hyperarousal of the motor cortex (and reward seeking circuits in the striatum) come with rhythmic exercise and externalization of rewards. To start, we need to consider the psychomotor circuitry involved in ADHD and other psychomotor issues, including OCD. Remember that just because a neural net is dominant, it doesn't mean it's functionally connected, which can lead to overexcitability issues.

Interestingly, ADHD is also known to involve the default mode network, where uncontrolled activity is thought to disrupt the frontoparietal control network (FPCN), which leads to attentional lapses. One of the major nodes of the default mode network (DMN) is the posterior cingulate cortex (PCC), which is considered dysfunctional in ADHD. In one study of almost four hundred patients with ADHD, the activity of the left PCC was increased (Nakao et al., 2011). Besides the PCC, dorsal ACC dysfunction has also been associated with inattention and impulsivity in ADHD (Bush et al., 1999).

The neural circuits that may need to be more functionally connected are likely the cerebellum, the anterior cingulate cortex (ACC), the posterior cingulate cortex, the corpus striatum, and the frontal and prefrontal regions. Translating this into neural networks, we can look at improving connectivity from the prefrontal (PF1, PF2) and frontal (F3, F4) regions for greater top down control over the limbic regions L1, L2, L3 and L4. We can also improve proprioceptive regions of the brain (P3, P4).

Prefrontal Regions 1 and 2
PF1 and PF2 (the higher prefrontal regions, including the orbitofrontal cortex (OFC) and medial prefrontal cortex (mPFC)) send dense inhibitory projections to the lower limbic regions, including the basal ganglia, in order to control excessive motor activity.

Frontal Regions 3 and 4
F3 is considered the seat of planning, sustained attention and working memory. F4 is responsive to tactile stimuli, visual stimuli and auditory stimuli. This region is also involved with inhibition of responses, maintaining motor coordination, verbal reasoning and problem solving. This same part of the brain is also associated with social and emotional judgment and planning.

Parietal Regions 3 and 4
P3 is part of the mirror neuron system and is involved in copying emotional tones, innuendo, nuance and non-verbal memory. It also has to do with identifying objects, symbol recognition, rote math, reading, spelling, cognitive reasoning, attention, short-term memory and imagination. P4 is the site related to proprioception that allows us to sense ourselves in space. P4 is also involved in visuomotor control, or directing attention, as well as maintaining an alert state.

Limbic Regions 1, 2, 3 and 4

L1 has to do with regulation of the body, senses, emotions and social ability. L2 is related to cognitive, motor and emotional regulation. L3 is related to regulation of unconscious fear memories. L4 has to do with cognitive, sensory-motor and emotional regulation.

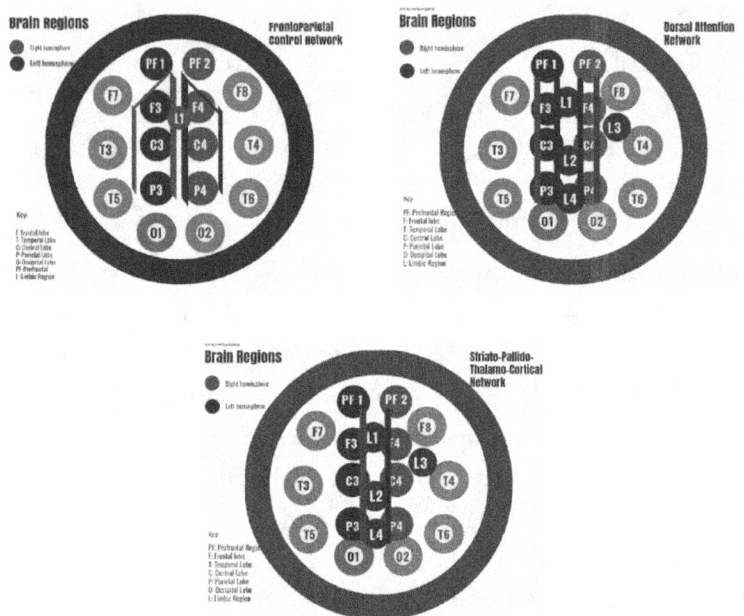

Improving prefrontal control over the limbic and motor cortex is the key to regulating psychomotor overexcitabilities. This can be initiated with motor activities and goal setting. With exercise, you are aiming to improve oxygenation and firing in the cerebellum and prefrontal cortex. This can balance out an asynchronous motor cortex and lead to better left-right hemispheric balance. In goal setting, we are externalizing working memory. In giving rewards, we are meeting the underlying need of the limbic brain. Essentially, we are looking at switching to and improving the function of the frontoparietal control network (FPCN) for reappraisal and intention setting, the dorsal attention network (DAN) for sustained attention, along with the striato-pallido-thalamo-cortical-network (SPTCN) for extinction learning.

According to Dr. Robert Melillo, founder of Brain Balance Centers, the key to functional integration is to improve everything from gross motor, fine motor, rhythm and timing, proprioception, visual and auditory processing, touch processing and cognitive skills. Gently stimulating the vestibular (inner ear) system can also add to hemispheric balance. Vestibular exercises can include rocking in a hammock, yoga inversion postures and even dancing slowly and swaying the body.

Practicing all of these skills consistently goes a long way to increasing functional connectivity of all regions of the brain. You can also check for primitive reflexes that may need to be reintegrated (see primitive reflex section below). Exercises can be used until all neural hotspots have calmed down and activity appears more coordinated. Please see brain-based therapies below for more sensory-motor exercises that may apply. The following activities are recommended in **Dr. Melillo's Brain Balance program** (Brain Balance Centers, 2017).

Motor activities include everything that improves:
- Muscle tone, strength and coordination
- Rhythm and timing, e.g., with aerobics, dancing or swimming
- Proprioception and vestibular balance
- Primitive reflexes (see primitive reflex section below)
- Bilateral coordination

- Eye muscle coordination and balance e.g. with yoga eye exercises

Other tips for those with Psychomotor Intelligence that may help include:
- Allowing time before, during and after work for physical activity
- Learning relaxation techniques
- Noticing exhaustion or need for quiet time
- Avoiding activities that require long periods of sitting
- Planning time outs, with rewards

Things to Consider
Proprioception - Sense of Self in Space

The most overlooked aspect in rehabilitating the sensory system is the sixth sense, or, proprioception, i.e., how we sense-feel ourselves in space. Proprioception is the ability to use muscle control and balance to resist gravity. It is also the greatest sensory stimulus for brain growth because, unlike any other stimulation, it occurs 24/7.

People with poor spatial orientation have a hard time knowing where they are in space. They have poor body awareness and don't feel grounded. As a result, they are unable to feel their bodies very well. People familiar with this feel that they never had good balance or they tend to feel "disconnected" to their limbs. If you don't feel your body well in space, you can't recognize your body and you don't have a good sense of yourself, which is the main problem to start correcting.

Once we get better at this skill of sensing ourself in space, we may be more adept at understanding our emotions, the emotions of others, and then more empathic social skills will likely be a side benefit. The remedy is to reboot our ability to perceive ourselves in space not only with brain balancing exercises but also with other sensory regulating activities. The invisible sense of proprioception can be improved with any of the rhythmic activities, martial arts, yoga and newer techniques like Feldenkrais. We can also use a body sock or weighted blankets when we feel overloaded.

Cerebellar Balance

The cerebellum is involved in many tasks and is essential for integrating balance centers and coordinating muscle activity. Importantly, studies are beginning to find that the massive streams of information pouring into the cerebellum from the cortex are processed and then redirected to many areas of the brain, appearing to coordinate complex mental as well as motor processes, including the allocation of attention and problem-solving functions (Allen et al., 1997). Interestingly, some studies have demonstrated that the posterior lobules of the cerebellum are involved in processes associated with cognitive and emotional functions (Depping et al., 2016). However, in those with depression, there may be a lack of segregation of emotional processing from cognitive and sensory-motor functions (Epstein et al., 2011). Supporting the cerebellum includes doing any rhythmic exercises and using balance boards. Please also review brain-based therapies below.

Target Brain Areas

Here is a summary chart to simplify all the information that we have covered so far.

Intelligence = Functional Integration	Disruptive Tendency	Potential Misdiagnosis	Brain Structures	Neuro-transmitters	Dominant Neural Nets	Brain Networks
	Intellectual Overexcitability	Depression Anxiety Rumination Allergies Autoimmune Disease ADHD	Dorsolateral PFC Posterior Parietal Cortex	Acetylcholine Serotonin Dopamine GABA	PF1, F3, F4, P3, P4	Central Executive Network (CEN)
	Emotional Overexcitability	ACE (Adverse Childhood Experiences) PTSD Anxiety Depression Rumination	Ventromedial Prefrontal Cortex Posterior Cingulate Cortex Anterior Cingulate Cortex Amygdala Hippocampus Anterior Insular Cortex	Serotonin Dopamine GABA	L1, L2, L3, L4	Default Mode Network (DMN) Salience Network (SN) Hypothalamic-Pituitary-Adrenal-Axis (HPA)
	Imaginational Overexcitability	Anxiety Depression Rumination Negativity Cluster B NPD BPD Histrionic Anti-social	Ventromedial Prefrontal Cortex Posterior Cingulate Cortex Amygdala Hippocampus Anterior Insular Cortex Anterior Insular Cortex	Serotonin Dopamine GABA	PF2, L3	Default Mode Network (DMN) Salience Network (SN) Hypothalamic-Pituitary-Adrenal-Axis (HPA)
	Psychomotor Overexcitability	ADHD, ADD, OCD	Basal Ganglia Motor Cortex Premotor Cortex Somatosensory Cortex Parietal Cortex Cerebellum Posterior Cingulate Cortex	Dopamine	F3, F4, P3, P4, C3, C4	Striato-Pallido-Thalamo-Cortical Network (SPTCN) Default Mode Network (DMN)
	Sensual Overexcitability	HSP, SPD Sensory Processing Sensitivity Environmental Sensitivity	Somatosensory Cortex Thalamus Anterior Insular Cortex Anterior Cingulate Cortex Bilateral Temporal, Medial and Posterior Parietal Regions Occipitotemporal Regions Cerebellum	Serotonin Dopamine GABA	C3, C4 F7, F8, P3, P4, T3, T4, T5, T6, O1, O2, L1, L2, L3, L4	Salience Network (SN) Hypothalamic-Pituitary-Adrenal-Axis (HPA)

Misdiagnosing Gifted Individuals

The problem with psychology and the healing arts professions is that, while practitioners can give good advice as to our personality needs, they're not going to be encouraging us to change our brain with neuroplastic techniques, simply because they have not yet studied this. Also, because there are so few mental health professionals who understand how giftedness impacts one's psychology, many gifted people are misdiagnosed with mood or personality disorders (Beduna et al., 2015).

People born with emotional intensity who are also highly perceptive, sensitive and intuitive may not yet know how to use their powerful gifts and live a more fulfilling life with increased self-knowledge. For this to occur, we need to learn what our gifts are and train ourselves with emotional regulation and self-regulation skills.

ANNE ANGELONE

Humanistic Psychology

One of the main functions of psychology is that it gives us the space to contemplate what it feels like just to be a human being. The reason to do psychotherapy in the first place is to relieve us of the burden of all the psychic contents that keep us from feeling our birthright, which is the experience of being-ness itself.

Humanistic psychology believes in the development of human potential and the understanding of life as a process where change is inevitable. This branch of psychological study takes the position that giftedness is not a pathology. From its perspective, our dominant neural circuits may be thought of as seeds of a super-perceptive level of emotional and moral development; they act as windows into the interior life of the gifted brain.

The Pre-History of Neuroplasticity and Psychology

It is a fact that the beginnings of psychoanalysis were nothing other than the scientific rediscovery of an ancient truth (Jung, 1933).

The main influences on the development of a 5Q Gifted Intelligence model includes Jung's personality psychology, Dabrowski's model of overexcitabilities as well as Taoist principles and the Yoga Sutras (teachings). If you think about it, the successful practice of psychology and neuroplasticity was first discovered thousands of years ago by Vedic yogis and Taoist sages - which explains why systems such as Tai Chi and acupuncture, along with Yoga, have been around for millennia. It has taken humanity a long time to understand these concepts and even longer to embody and retain these principles. Yet, these are the current principles of functional integration that were presaged and practiced by the ancients - way before Neuroscience, Dabrowski or Carl Jung hit the map.

It seems that Taoist concepts of Yin-Yang, acupuncture, 5-Element personality theory and Yoga precepts along with Carl Jung and Dabrowski's ideas about personality type, laid the foundation for neuroscience to discover brain regions and neural networks related to the psyche that we continue to learn about today.

Jungian Psychology and Individuation

Many personality type tests are based on Carl Jung's landmark ideas about cognitive processes. Like Dabrowski, Carl Jung was deeply interested in the development of the human psyche. In his book, *Psychological Types*, Jung developed the theory of cognitive processes (mental functions) that are characterized as preferential ways of perceiving and judging, i.e., thinking, feeling, sensation and intuition.

Carl Jung thought it was possible to attain complete knowledge of the Self but that it would take a lot of inner work. Individuation for Jung meant becoming an individual through acceptance of our dominant cognitive preferences, and their shadow (the parts we are unaware of).

In the 5Q model, we can now look at Jung's ideas through the new lens of dominant neural networks for each preference. For example, thinking, perceiving and judging have to do with the default mode network (DMN), the central executive network (CEN) and the frontoparietal control network (FPCN), while intuiting, sensing and feeling are handled by the salience network (SN).

Finally, when you study the Yogic Sutras, you learn that our psychic nature includes all of the same intelligences that are included in this model. That is, our cognitive, emotional, sensory, motor and intuitive processes are considered contents of the psyche. This may be likened to functional integration leading to the prized human ability to use brain networks involved in metacognition as well as moral cognition or ethics – all made possible by the FPCN.

We can now think of the psyche as neural patterns spread throughout our brain. Our personality, used to express our psychic nature, can now be seen as brain processes that represent dominant patterns of functioning. These are the fundamental neural nets that animate the life of the gifted. Once we learn about the contents of our psychic self, we can recognize our transcendent nature. This is the same as the process of transformation, individuation and self-realization.

Neurospsychology, Functional Connectivity and Personality

From the viewpoint of neuroscience, our symptoms reflect our preset neurobiology and downstream emotional, creative and behavioral styles. They exemplify aspects of our psychical nature that are calling our attention to personality development.

Having studied and practiced Chinese medicine for over twenty-five years, I am trained to pick up on 5-Element personality types and tendencies as a way to track people's psychological tendencies through the physical traces of their illness. This "Inner Tradition" of Chinese Medicine holds out a similar process of individuation and personality development as the yogis, the Taoists, Jung and Dabrowski. The general theory is that adversity brings learning and knowledge, but it doesn't guarantee wisdom and freedom of distress and disease. Because of the nature of our human drives, this will be an intentional process that we need to choose.

Once we achieve individuation, we can leave the model behind and move on to spiritual intelligence or connection to universal consciousness and the unified field. This state of consciousness recruits all regions of the brain and is referred to as the numinous brain network.

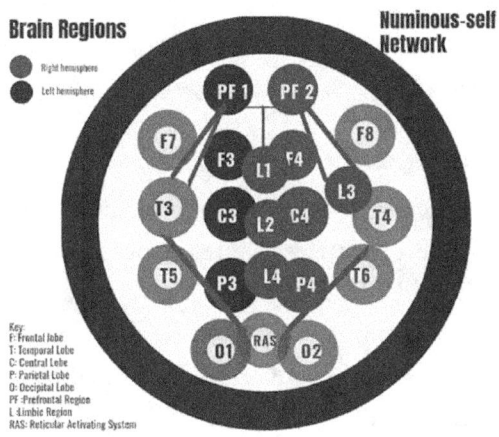

The ultimate goal is recognizing when our brain states are either expansive – as in the FPCN brain state – or contractive as in the DMN. Having a deeper understanding of our brain states makes it easier to shift them as needed.

The 5Q Model of Individuation

To have agency in our lives, we must understand and master the flow of information streaming through our brains and be able to assess whether this flow is expressing smoothly or not. In the 5Q model, we can describe our personality as made up of IQ, EQ, NQ, PQ and SQ. Consider each quality of intelligence as a functionally connected neural network. Ultimately, it's about supporting the brain to integrate sensory, emotional and cognitive data by improving hemispheric balance. When the hemispheres are balanced, this is called functional integration. In the 5Q model, we can initiate and lock in the psycho-neuro-immuno-sensory-behavioral plasticity that we need, and know exactly what to do when we start falling off the mark of what feels like normal brain balance. While overexcitabilities are rooted in dominant neural nets that may or may not be functionally connected, intelligence represents the developmental potential of our personalities as networks become more functionally connected. This leads to a new neurobiological understanding of both personality and individuation.

In the 5Q model, we can say that individuation is a process of transformation whereby the all intelligences are brought into consciousness (e.g., by means of symptoms, assessments and treatments), to be assimilated into the whole personality. The ultimate goal is to build functional connectivity and yield hemispheric balance. The task is to use novel modalities to stimulate stable wiring in brain regions that need it most.

This means that if, for example, you're very sensitive, you can help yourself become more balanced by working on neuroplasticity. This can be accomplished by accessing the parasympathetic nervous system and the sensory processing areas in critical systems like the olfactory, vestibular, proprioceptive, visual, auditory, limbic, temporal, parietal and occipital regions. You can support these systems with essential oils, balance exercises and sound/music therapy that is comforting and satisfying. In this way, you can work on the underlying causes of these brain-based imbalances that are manifesting as behavioral tendencies or other symptoms.

The takeaway is that we can improve functional connectivity with precise stimulation to boost accurate intelligence. We can consider that, from a neurobiological perspective, hyper and hypo-connectivity in these areas go hand-in-hand with symptom manifestation. However, with the goal of changing the organization of our neural circuitry, we will be able to change our immune system and inflammatory responses directly from the nervous system. This process is facilitated by neuroplastic exercises.

At the end of the day, people want to know themselves better. If the ultimate goal of individuation is to reintegrate all parts of your personality by improving functional connectivity, you will be much more self-aware and fulfilled in life. There is a deeper part of you that is waiting to be discovered and integrated.

Understanding our dominant neural nets can be likened to understanding the universal blueprints or deeper potentialities of our own individuation and those of others. Considering the developmental potential for each aspect of intelligence provides the opportunity to reflect on our own individuation and psychological maturation processes, where we integrate all aspects of our personality including sensory, psychomotor, emotional, intuitive and cognitive intelligence.

Brain-Based Therapies

The foundation of neuroplasticity starts with precise sensory and motor interaction with the environment. If we did not get adequate or correct stimulation, we may be at a loss of full function. Yet even with the hope of neuroplasticity, we can't forget the fact that once neurons die, they die. The good news is that you can increase the functional connectivity *around* these non-functioning neurons to *other* neurons, which builds up networks and improved structural flow. This is what we're looking to do when we talk about improving the functional connectivity of the brain.

The bottom line is that the brain can change, but neuroplasticity is not a fool's errand - it requires intention and dogged application. It requires agency, perhaps a little guidance, and a lot of practice for recovery of your sense of self.

Secrets to Improving Sensory-Motor Intelligence

Movement and sensory exploration can be traced back from the activity of our mitochondria and immune cells all the way through to the evolution of the sensory-motor functions of the cerebellum and cerebral cortex. From a functional neurobiology standpoint, it is crucial to improve motor skills along with sensory processing for neuroplasticity (and immune balance) to occur. From the point of view of sensory processing, the goal is to strengthen the integrity of connections in the sensory structures of the brain along with motor function.

It has been said that movement is like nutrition for the brain. Functional disconnection (loss of connectivity among brain networks) occurs because timing and coordination is off in the motor system. The functional neurology approach is to steadily apply brain-balancing movements to improve the ability to learn, focus, pay attention and regulate emotions. Since coordination and timing are key to getting the brain to work properly, rhythmic movement is your best bet for functional connectivity.

Movement allows us to engage our senses via the cerebellum, somatosensory cortex and thalamus. By activating proprioception and vestibular balance, multiple areas of the brain start working simultaneously to improve connectivity through rhythm and timing. Rhythmic movement also leads to decreased hyperarousal of the sympathetic nervous system, improved muscle tone and a change in the way the body responds to stimuli, which ultimately supports immune balance.

Give the Brain What it Craves
Start by recognizing brain connectivity patterns that can be tuned up or down, depending on the desired effect. Then supply the precise inputs with adequate frequency and duration. The following practices can be used to maximize sensory-motor awareness, which will set the foundation of self-care in terms of maximizing the brain's most craved sensory inputs.

Weighted Blankets
Weighted blankets are sensory tools that were traditionally used by occupational therapists to help bring calm to children with ADHD, SPD and autism spectrum disorders. These days, weighted blankets are marketed to people with anxiety and insomnia who benefit from being comfortably weighed down and snuggled in by gravity.

The therapeutic effect from deep pressure due to the weight causes the body to produce serotonin and endorphins, which are the chemicals our bodies naturally use to feel relaxed or calm. The weight is intended to provide proprioceptive input to the brain, which has a calming and organizing effect on the central nervous system.

Body Socks

A body sock is a therapeutic modality used in occupational therapy to address deficits in proprioception, endurance and body awareness. By stretching in a body-size sock, a person triggers deep proprioceptive input to the muscles and joints. This in turn provides an outlet for sensory seeking and self-stimming to balance sympathetic arousal and tension in the body.

Posture and proprioception are linked to the vestibular (inner-ear) system and oculomotor system. Training proprioception and vestibular input improves our sense of balance and movement, which in turn improves body awareness.

Using a body sock also increases endurance because you are working against the resistance of the material. While you stretch and pull the sock, pay attention to the feedback about where your body parts are in relation to one another in the sock.

Sound and Music Therapy to Improve the Connectome

Neuroscience has proven (through functional brain imaging) that when we listen to music, virtually the whole brain lights up. Music listening not only involves the auditory areas of the brain, but also engages large-scale neural networks, including the prefrontal cortex, motor cortex, sensory cortex, visual cortex, cerebellum, hippocampus, amygdala, nucleus accumbens, corpus callosum, autonomic nervous system, vestibular system and the enteric nervous system.

Sound and music therapy connects the most ancient parts of the brain (the brainstem and limbic-emotional brain) to the most advanced prefrontal cortex, or, our social brain. Binaural beats are also used for building new brain connections between the right and left hemispheres of our brain by optimizing frequencies such as alpha, theta and delta.

Benefits include greater mental clarity, improved memory and immune balance. Listening can be a daily practice to help with autism, reading, learning, attention, sensory processing and autoimmune flares. You can add sound and music therapies based on the part of the brain that needs it most. For example, a person who has a highly reactive amygdala would do well with calming instrumental music, nature sounds, or Tibetan bowls to relax.

The way to listen is to sit or lie comfortably, close your eyes and breathe slowly and deeply. For maximum long term benefits, listen daily for a period of six weeks and then as needed. I have created an Autoimmune Brain Balance program in my studio for this express purpose; they are available for review <u>on my website</u>.

Emo-Sensory Therapy
With Emo-Sensory Therapy, the goal is to experience sound on a tactile level, where you are immersed in a 3D soundscape that is deeply therapeutic. The selections are designed to support specific regions of the brain. To support hemispheric balance, I use meditation bowls for creating a steady binaural backdrop to each 3D soundscape. You can review Emo-Sensory Therapy mp3s <u>on my website</u>.

Essential Oils
The benefits of essential oil therapy include reducing sympathetic nervous system activity and inducing the relaxation response, which in turn benefits the immune system. Essential oil benefits are largely due to the inhalation of terpenes which are the volatile oils found in many plants. These terpenes have been shown to

exhibit strong biological activity on many systems, including the brain and immune system. Essential oils can also decrease anxiety, depression, anger, fatigue and confusion.

Given that therapeutic terpenes like pinene, myrcene and limonene are important for decreasing inflammation, calming the mind and creating immune balance, you can also consider diffusing the essential oils of pine, citrus, and lavender in your own home. Pine is high in pinene (known to improve mental clarity), citrus is high in limonene (which uplifts our mood) and lavender is high in myrcene (which calms anxiety). For more information about essential oils blends for immune balance, please read my guide, *Beyond Cannabis*.

Optimizing Self-Regulation

Self-regulation refers to willfully managing our impulses to stay in line with our life goals. Gifted individuals need a comprehensive method for self-regulation. They personally know that lack of self-regulation can lead to increased sensitivities, depression, anxiety, ADHD, OCD and autoimmune reactions. They need a variety of tools that support the regulation of thoughts, feelings, sensations and behavior.

When you have an under-functioning prefrontal cortex and poor executive control, you likely need help managing thoughts, feelings, behaviors and symptoms. Here's where a combination of neuroplastic techniques and sensory-motor therapies may be very helpful.

Many cognitive-behavioral therapists focus on using top-down cognitive means of self-regulation, such as cognitive reappraisal, reframing and goal setting. While sensory-motor exercises represent a bottom-up approach (from the body to the brain), top-down strategies are practiced by putting an emphasis on attentional control, and thus, top-down executive mechanisms from brain to body (Gard et al., 2014). Some of the most powerful methods of top-down self-regulation include meditation and mindfulness.

Meditation and Mindfulness

Humanity has only recently become conscious of how to use the prefrontal cortex for emotional regulation. While Buddhists and yogis have been teaching emotional and self-regulation skills, e.g., meditation, pratyahara (withdrawal of the senses and interoception), asanas (yoga postures) and breathing techniques (pranayama) for millennia, it's only been in the past 40 years that we in the West have been turning our attention to these powerful introspective technologies, which stem from these teachings.

Mindfulness is basically applied self-awareness. Mindfulness helps us stay more in touch with our intuition and body messages. We can use it to monitor signals from our own bodies as a way to develop a deeper sense of non-verbal body wisdom, which does not come from thought. That is, we become more adept at using the salience network. Dogged practice changes the nature of self-referencing, detachment from self-concept and perceived fear by altering the function and activity of the default mode network. Remember that the default network is a set of brain regions that activate when we are engaged in mind wandering, daydreaming and imagining. Meditation involves training the brain over and over to maintain attention and focus on consciousness itself and to have more primed, open awareness. This also helps us shift out of the default mode network and into metacognition made possible by the frontoparietal control network (FPCN).

Clinically, mindfulness and meditation practices have proven beneficial for the treatment of chronic pain, depression and have contributed to an increase in general well-being. The American Psychological Association lists, amongst many other benefits, reduced rumination and stress reduction as results of mindfulness practice. In 2010, Hoffman et al. reviewed thirty-nine papers that found meditation practitioners experience less neural reactivity to stressful stimuli, less anxiety and depressive ideation, along with greater attentional focus. This in turn benefits the immune system.

Yogic Breathing Techniques - Pranayama
The science behind pranayama (the building of life force through specific breathing techniques) shows that these exercises release neuropeptides from the lungs that, by way of the cerebrospinal fluid, reach the periaqueductal gray area of the midbrain. This is a key nodal point that releases natural opiates. This is likely one of the reasons (besides hemispheric balance) why yogic breathing techniques are thought to be very helpful for pain, depression and anxiety. To learn more about meditation and pranayama, check out my classes on my website.

Primitive Reflexes
Finally, it's important to know about primitive reflexes, since it is thought that overexcitabilities may be rooted in reflexes that have not yet been integrated. These include the spinal gallant, fear paralysis and Moro reflexes. Integration of these primitive reflexes may be a great self-help practice for decreasing hyperarousal states that tend to come with overexcitabilities.

Primitive reflexes originate in the brain stem – the brain area that is responsible for survival. As we get older, unintegrated reflexes can interfere with neurological organization and may trigger a chronic flight/flight response, challenges with coordination, reading and writing difficulties, language and speech delays, disorganization, fidgeting and concentration problems.

Unintegrated, active primitive reflexes may be caused by breech birth, birth trauma, caesarean birth and/or lack of proper movement in infancy which delays brain development. Other things that can trigger unintegrated reflexes include illness, trauma, injury, chronic stress, environmental toxins, dietary imbalances or sensitivities. Because primitive reflexes start at the base of the brain, functions that develop above them may not wire properly which can contribute to:

- Hemispheric Imbalance
- Autism Spectrum Disorders
- Sensory Disorders
- Hyperactivity
- ADHD
- Speech Disorders
- Social Disorders
- Asthma
- Dyslexia
- Dysgraphia
- Dyscalculia
- Immune Disorders

Primitive reflexes can be restored with simple brain balance exercises, which are briefly described below.

Fear Paralysis Reflex (FPR)
The FPR is a withdrawal reflex to stress that starts in utero. If this reflex is retained it may lead to symptoms of withdrawal, fear of

new situations and a tendency towards negativity. This is an avoidance tactic referred to as "the freeze response," which is regulated in the medulla by the vagus nerve. Since many of these symptoms overlap with autoimmune, sensory processing, behavior and learning disorders, it's important not to overlook the fact that you can still improve or reintegrate these reflexes if needed. Fill out the following questionnaire to see if this applies to you.

Retained Fear Paralysis Reflex

Retained Fear Paralysis Reflex Questionnaire	YES	NO
Shallow, difficult breathing	☐	☐
Underlying anxiety or negativity	☐	☐
Insecure, low self-esteem	☐	☐
Depression/isolation/withdrawal	☐	☐
Constant feelings of overwhelm	☐	☐
Extreme shyness, fear in groups	☐	☐
Excessive fear of embarrassment	☐	☐
Fear of separation from a loved one, clinging	☐	☐
Sleep & eating disorders	☐	☐
Feeling stuck	☐	☐
Withdrawal from touch	☐	☐
Extreme fear of failure, perfectionism	☐	☐
Phobias	☐	☐
Aggressive or controlling behavior	☐	☐
Low tolerance to stress	☐	☐

If any of these symptoms relate to you, you can start with a simple exercise to reintegrate the Fear Paralysis Reflex. To reintegrate the FPR, you can do a restorative yoga posture, which simply requires you to lie back on a bolster or supportive pillow, spread your arms out wide and open your chest. Do this for at least five minutes, twice a day, until the reflex goes away.

This helps decrease hyperarousal of the sympathetic nervous system and reintegrate the FPR.

Moro Reflex, aka the Startle Reflex

It is common to find an active FPR in tandem with an unintegrated Moro reflex. The Moro Reflex, aka the Startle Reflex, is an automatic response to a sudden change in sensory stimuli (bright light, change in body position, temperature, loud noise, intense touch, etc.). This may stem from birth trauma. If left unintegrated, this can trigger a chronic fight-flight response along with sensory processing and learning problems. Since many of these symptoms overlap with autoimmune, sensory processing, behavior and learning disorders, it's important not to overlook the fact that you can still improve or reintegrate these reflexes if needed.

Moro Reflex Test and Starfish Exercises

To test for the Moro reflex, lie on your back and spread your arms and legs out wide, starfish style. Then, bring your arms and legs in, crossing your arms over your chest, and crossing your legs one over the other, keeping them straight in the lying down position, comfortably. Notice which arm and leg are on top. Now spread your arms and legs out wide again, then bring them in again, this time with the right leg and right arm on top. Repeat with left arm and left leg on top. If crossing right and left gets confusing, the reflex is still present and needs to be integrated with these same "Starfish Exercises" (Boss, 2017). Repeat for five minutes, twice a day, until the reflex goes away.

GIFTED INTELLIGENCE

Fill out the following questionnaire to see if this applies to you.

Retained Moro Reflex Symptom Questionnaire	YES	NO
Easily triggered, reacts in anger or emotional outbursts	☐	☐
Poor balance and coordination	☐	☐
Poor stamina	☐	☐
Poor digestion, tendency towards hypoglycemia	☐	☐
Weak immune system; asthma, allergies and infections	☐	☐
Hypersensitivity to light, movement, sound, touch & smell	☐	☐
Vision/reading/writing difficulties	☐	☐
Difficulty adapting to change	☐	☐
Cycles of hyperactivity and extreme fatigue	☐	☐
Frequently in the "fight or flight" mode; always on edge; heightened state of awareness	☐	☐
Anxiety	☐	☐
Exaggerated startle reaction	☐	☐
Motion sickness	☐	☐
Poor impulse control	☐	☐
Mood swings	☐	☐

Spinal Galant Reflex

The Spinal Galant Reflex is thought to help balance and coordination and may be present in those with asynchronous PFC/motor cortices, e.g., ADHD and other psychomotor issues - see checklist below. Since many of these symptoms overlap with autoimmune, sensory processing, learning and behavior disorders, it's important not to overlook the fact that you can still improve or reintegrate these reflexes.

Consider reintegrating this reflex if any of the following are still an issue.

Unintegrated Spinal Galant Reflex Questionnaire	YES	NO
Fidgeting/hyperactivity	☐	☐
Poor short-term memory	☐	☐
Poor posture	☐	☐
Poor coordination	☐	☐
Poor concentration	☐	☐
Poor endurance	☐	☐
Attention difficulties	☐	☐
Hip rotation to one side/scoliosis	☐	☐

Spinal Galant Test

To test the Spinal Galant Reflex, just lightly stroke down each side of the lower spine. You can tell that the reflex is still present if either side twitches. If so, you can do the following snow angel exercises twice daily for five minutes until the reflex goes away.

Snow Angels
Anyone who grew up with snowy winters can remember making snow angels. It turns out that this is a great exercise to reintegrate the Spinal Galant Reflex. You can pretend it's snowing anytime, anywhere. Lie down on the floor or on a mat and open your arms and legs wide. Then bring your arms down to your sides while you move your legs close together. Then open up your arms and legs again to the wide position. Repeat for five minutes, twice a day, until the reflex goes away.

Anti-inflammatory Diet Basics
Because gifted brains tend to have one or more highly charged neural circuits, the chances of brain inflammation may be higher. Also, some may suffer with food allergies along with a leaky gut, and would do well with an anti-inflammatory diet.

Although anti-inflammatory diets vary, there are some basics to follow:

Eliminate all processed foods, fast foods, desserts, sodas, etc. These foods are designed to be addictive. Your anti-inflammatory diet should consist mainly of whole foods found in the produce and meat sections of the grocery store, with an emphasis on plenty of vegetables. Also, eliminate processed vegetable oils and hydrogenated oils. Stick with natural oils such as coconut oil and olive oil.

Eliminate common inflammatory foods. The most common culprit is gluten, the protein found in wheat, rye, barley, and other wheat-like grains. However, you may have developed an intolerance to other foods, including dairy, eggs, soy, and nuts. Eliminate these foods for about a month to see whether you react upon reintroducing them one at a time.

On the anti-inflammatory diet, you avoid all sweeteners, including excessive amounts of natural ones such as honey and maple syrup. This helps curb cravings, stabilize blood sugar and lower inflammation. Enjoy fruit instead, such as berries.

Some people may need to follow stricter versions of this diet, such as in, *The Autoimmune Diet*, one of my publications, which describes the importance of eliminating grains, foods with lectins and nightshades. An anti-inflammatory diet can be tailored to individual needs, but the focus is on clearing out the junk and getting back to foods in their most natural state, with an emphasis on plenty of leafy green vegetables. I have also found that adding nutritional compounds to repair a leaky gut and faulty methylation (when appropriate) adds to the powerful effects of an anti-inflammatory diet.

Dietary Support for Environmental Sensitivities

Since so many people notice feeling worse when exposed to environmental and chemical sensitivities, it's important to know how to protect yourself. Environmental and chemical sensitivities are now called TILT (toxicant-induced loss of tolerance). TILT happens when the body loses the ability to tolerate environmental compounds such as:

- Artificial chemicals and preservatives in food
- Pharmaceuticals

- Gas fumes/exhaust, scented body products, cleaning supplies, laundry products, new car or carpeting smells, pesticides and fertilizers.

Besides a right hemisphere weakness, other causes of TILT include depletion or poor absorption of glutathione and Vitamin D, and omega-3 fatty acid deficiency, along with high amounts of stress and chronic inflammation.

Besides decreasing stress and getting your vitamin D level checked, you can add omega 3 fats with extra fish oils by taking supplements and/or by eating fish high in omega 3s such as salmon. You can also start increasing glutathione levels naturally with sulfur rich vegetables such as cauliflower, watercress, garlic, onions, broccoli, kale, collards, cabbage and scallions. Supplements that specifically support glutathione include N-acetyl-cysteine, alpha lipoic acid, selenium, milk thistle (silymarin), gotu kola, and S-acetyl-glutathione or liposomal glutathione.

The Gifted Brain Mood and Personality Questionnaire

About the Questionnaire:

I have created a Gifted Brain Mood and Personality Questionnaire (GBMAPQ) specifically for those of us who have autoimmune, mood, sensory, learning and/or behavioral issues. The questionnaire also explores the aging process in the brain and neurodegenerative symptoms. Losses of function, such as memory, balance, hearing, creativity, motivation, social skills, cognitive, emotional and sensory integration will be assessed.
The GBMAPQ is a quick and effective way to determine strategies to support brain health. This process is used to help formulate effective dietary, nutritional and brain-based approaches. It is not

used to identify or diagnose any diseases of the brain or personality disorders.

I've sorted the questionnaire into sections related to general brain health, hemispheric balance, overexcitabilities, primitive reflexes and need for neurotransmitters.

Remember that, as in any system, it is sometimes difficult to classify a person as a single type. There are many different moods, attitudes, behaviors and actions considered that may not all fit into one category, and you may find yourself noticing you have more Yes or No answers in a particular section. Use this new data to inform brain health, hemispheric balance and increased awareness of your dominant functions.

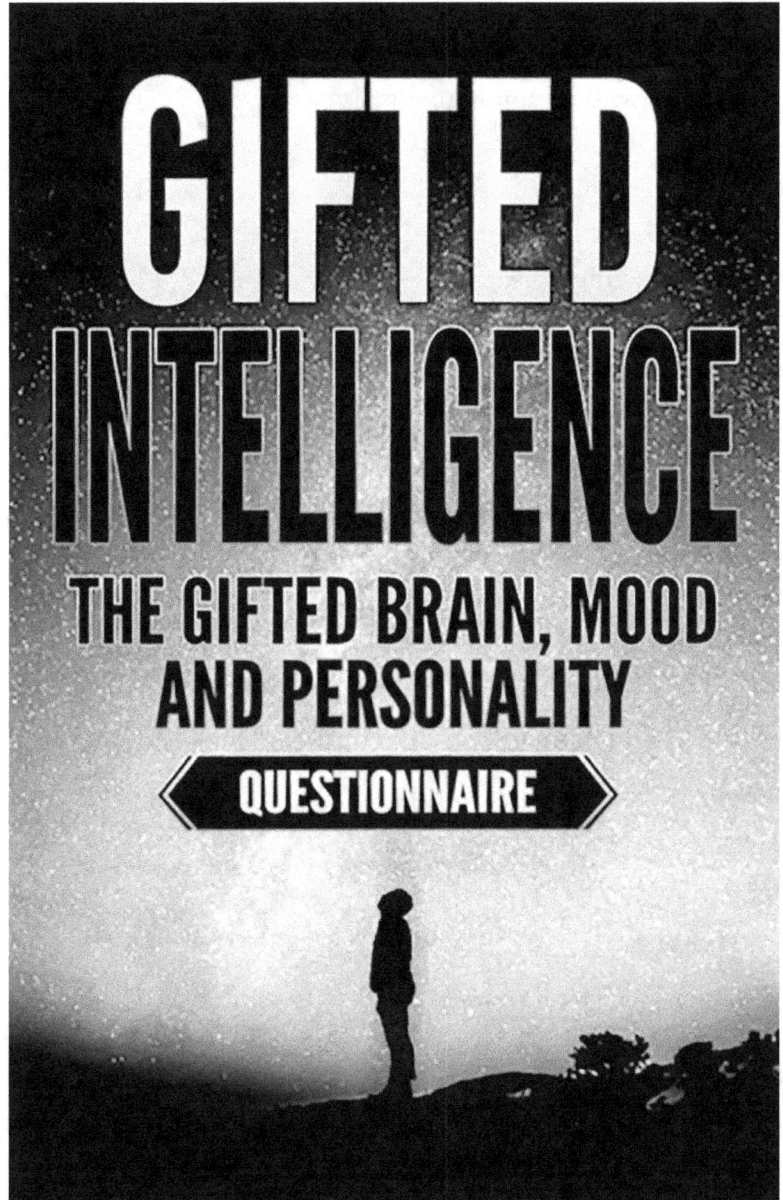

SECTION 1 GENERAL SCREENING   YES   NO

	YES	NO
Diagnosed with an autoimmune disease	☐	☐
Food sensitivities	☐	☐
Asthma	☐	☐
ADHD	☐	☐
Autism Spectrum Disorder	☐	☐
Fibromyalgia	☐	☐
Environmental sensitivities	☐	☐
Emotionally anxious	☐	☐
Emotionally depressed	☐	☐
Emotionally compulsive	☐	☐
Irritable Bowel Syndrome	☐	☐
Eczema	☐	☐
Poor sense of body in space	☐	☐
Rapid heartbeat and/or high blood pressure	☐	☐
Sensory Processing Disorder or Sensitivities	☐	☐

SECTION 2 BRAIN HEALTH   YES   NO

	YES	NO
Inability to concentrate	☐	☐
Difficulty planning or problem solving	☐	☐
Cold hands and feet	☐	☐
Frequent memory lapses	☐	☐
Decreased sense of smell	☐	☐
Difficulty sleeping	☐	☐
Episodes of dizziness or light-headedness	☐	☐
Brain fog (unclear thoughts or concentration)	☐	☐
Constipation or irregular bowel movements	☐	☐
Difficulty swallowing supplements	☐	☐
Difficulty with balance	☐	☐
Difficulty with right/left discrimination	☐	☐
Poor handwriting	☐	☐
Reduced function in overall hearing	☐	☐
Difficulty recognizing symbols, words, letters	☐	☐

SECTION 3 INTELLECTUAL OVEREXCITABILITY

	YES	NO
Very curious and freely approaches new situations	☐	☐
Highly verbal	☐	☐
Analytic thinker	☐	☐
Keen observer	☐	☐
Good at memorizing large amounts of data	☐	☐
Avid reader	☐	☐
Preoccupation with concepts	☐	☐
Detailed planner	☐	☐
Searches for truth and understanding	☐	☐
Perseveres in interests	☐	☐
Love of problem solving	☐	☐
Learns new things rapidly	☐	☐
Motivated by ideas	☐	☐
Asks probing questions	☐	☐
Good concentration and ability to maintain intellectual effort	☐	☐

SECTION 4 EMOTIONAL OVEREXCITABILITY

	YES	NO
Intense anger or problems controlling anger	☐	☐
Feelings of guilt and sense of responsibility	☐	☐
Inability to handle stress – easily overwhelmed	☐	☐
Identifies with the feelings of others	☐	☐
Feelings of inadequacy and inferiority	☐	☐
Anxiety	☐	☐
Depression	☐	☐
Very sensitive to criticism	☐	☐
Physical response to emotions (stomach aches, headaches)	☐	☐
Struggles with mood swings	☐	☐
Concerned with death	☐	☐
Strong somatic expressions – blushing, sweaty palms	☐	☐
Heightened sense of right and wrong, injustice and hypocrisy	☐	☐

SECTION 5 SENSUAL OVEREXCITABILITY

	YES	NO
Very perceptive and insightful	☐	☐
Delights in nature, beautiful objects, form and color	☐	☐
Delights in music and the sound of words	☐	☐
Enhanced sensory and aesthetic pleasure	☐	☐
Highly intuitive to others' feelings	☐	☐
Thin skinned or feels emotionally porous	☐	☐
Startles easily	☐	☐
Sensitive to perfumes, foods, alcohol, etc.	☐	☐
Thrives in an encouraging environment	☐	☐
Avoids negative and/or violent movies	☐	☐
Experiences sensory overload	☐	☐
Easily overwhelmed at parties or in large crowds	☐	☐
Easily bothered by noise, lights and smells	☐	☐
Dislikes words and events that hurt animals or people	☐	☐
Requires a large amount of downtime or alone time	☐	☐

SECTION 6 PSYCHOMOTOR OVEREXCITABILITY

	YES	NO
Rapid speech	☐	☐
Likes competition - thrives on challenges	☐	☐
Has issues with sleeplessness	☐	☐
Compulsive organizing	☐	☐
Fidgety – can't sit still	☐	☐
Feels out of step with others	☐	☐
Prefers fast action and sports	☐	☐
Nervous habits and tics	☐	☐
Workaholic	☐	☐
Marked excitation and acting out	☐	☐
Poor impulse control	☐	☐
Prefers intense physical activity	☐	☐
Hyperactive	☐	☐
Impatient and easily frustrated	☐	☐
Poor coordination	☐	☐

SECTION 7 IMAGINATIONAL OVEREXCITABILITY

	YES	NO
Loves symbolism and metaphors	☐	☐
Has a persistent curiosity	☐	☐
Has a good sense of humor	☐	☐
Engages in animistic and magical thinking	☐	☐
Has a love of poetry, music, drama	☐	☐
Has a facility for invention and fantasy	☐	☐
Has vivid dreams	☐	☐
Has a tendency to mix truth with fiction	☐	☐
Has a facility for detailed visualization and imagination	☐	☐
Uses intuition and hunches	☐	☐
Sees the big picture	☐	☐
Bored by routine	☐	☐
Can connect seemingly unrelated ideas	☐	☐
Has unusual ideas or perceptions	☐	☐
Acutely aware of own and others' feelings	☐	☐

SECTION 8 SEROTONIN   YES   NO

	YES	NO
Loss of pleasure in hobbies and interests	☐	☐
Has had bouts of depression	☐	☐
Struggles with feelings of sadness	☐	☐
Worries	☐	☐
Inability to fall into deep, restful sleep	☐	☐
Noticeable loss of enjoyment in life	☐	☐
Feelings of sadness in winter or in overcast weather	☐	☐
Loss of enthusiasm for favorite activities	☐	☐
Loss of enjoyment in friendships and relationships	☐	☐
Susceptible to pain – low pain threshold	☐	☐

SECTION 9 DOPAMINE   YES   NO

	YES	NO
Lack feelings of contentment	☐	☐
Desire to isolate from others	☐	☐
Chronic feelings of emptiness	☐	☐
Feelings of worthlessness	☐	☐
Feelings of hopelessness	☐	☐
Disinterest in hobbies, social activities or work	☐	☐
Anger and aggression when stressed	☐	☐
Unexplained lack of concern for family and friends	☐	☐
Inability to finish tasks	☐	☐
Feelings of tiredness even after a good night's rest	☐	☐

SECTION 10 GABA | YES | NO

	YES	NO
Feelings of nervousness or panic for no reason	☐	☐
Feelings of dread	☐	☐
Feelings of being overwhelmed for no reason	☐	☐
Feelings of guilt about everyday decisions	☐	☐
Restless mind	☐	☐
Inability to turn off the mind when relaxing	☐	☐
Disorganized attention	☐	☐
Feelings of inner tension	☐	☐
Low level anxiety	☐	☐
Seeks safety and security	☐	☐

SECTION 11 ACETYLCHOLINE · YES · NO

	YES	NO
Decrease in visual imagery (shapes and images)	☐	☐
Difficulty calculating numbers	☐	☐
Difficulty recognizing names and faces	☐	☐
Decrease in comprehension	☐	☐
Decrease in creativity	☐	☐
Occurrence of memory lapses	☐	☐
Disorganized attention	☐	☐
Difficulty finding words when speaking	☐	☐
Difficulty spelling familiar words	☐	☐
Difficulty with directions/maps	☐	☐

GIFTED INTELLIGENCE

SECTION 12 FEAR PARALYSIS RELFEX

	YES	NO
Shallow, difficult breathing	☐	☐
Underlying anxiety or negativity	☐	☐
Insecure, low self-esteem	☐	☐
Depression/isolation/withdrawal	☐	☐
Constant feelings of overwhelm	☐	☐
Extreme shyness, fear in groups	☐	☐
Excessive fear of embarrassment	☐	☐
Fear of separation from a loved one, clinging	☐	☐
Sleep & eating disorders	☐	☐
Feeling stuck	☐	☐
Withdrawal from touch	☐	☐
Extreme fear of failure, perfectionism	☐	☐
Phobias	☐	☐
Aggressive or controlling behavior	☐	☐
Low tolerance to stress	☐	☐

SECTION 13 RETAINED MORO RELFEX

	YES	NO
Easily triggered, reacts in anger or emotional outburst	☐	☐
Poor balance and coordination	☐	☐
Poor stamina	☐	☐
Poor digestion, tendency towards hypoglycemia	☐	☐
Weak immune system, asthma, allergies and infections	☐	☐
Hypersensitivity to light, movement, sound, touch and smell	☐	☐
Vision/reading/writing difficulties	☐	☐
Difficulty adapting to change	☐	☐
Cycles of hyperactivity and extreme fatigue	☐	☐
Frequently in the "fight or flight" mode; always on edge; heightened state of awareness	☐	☐
Anxiety	☐	☐
Exaggerated startle reaction	☐	☐
Motion sickness	☐	☐
Poor impulse control	☐	☐
Mood swings	☐	☐

SECTION 14 RETAINED SPINAL GALANT REFLEX   YES   NO

	YES	NO
Fidgeting/hyperactivity	☐	☐
Poor short-term memory	☐	☐
Poor posture	☐	☐
Poor coordination	☐	☐
Poor concentration	☐	☐
Poor endurance	☐	☐
Attention difficulties	☐	☐
Hip rotation to one side/scoliosis	☐	☐

Final Thoughts

Precise interventions for immune, sensory, learning, behavioral and mood disorders are an increasingly urgent concern in a world that lacks corresponding professional support for individuals who experience hypersensitive brain circuitry. Those with sensory, mood, immune and/or behavioral disorders may have multiple sensitivities that result from these highly sensitized brain circuits.

Understanding the five intelligences of the gifted brain are a means of connecting more deeply to the experiences many individuals have of life. This book lays the foundation for expanding research and clinical evaluation of people with a wide range of immune, emotional, learning, behavioral and sensory challenges.

I could not have conceived of this work were it not for my own experience with autoimmune disease as well as my background in music, yoga, meditation, Traditional Chinese and Functional Medicine. I have tremendous gratitude for all of the teachers and healers who have inspired me and hope that this work will be a guiding light to those who need it most.

Thank you for taking the time to read this book. If you are gifted, please remember that we were not meant to live an easily overwhelmed life. We are designed to live in harmony with our environment, to interact effectively with our fellow humans and live inspired lives.

To learn more about my work and projects, please check out my website.

References

Acevedo, et al. The highly sensitive brain: an fMRI study of sensory processing sensitivity and response to others' emotions. Brain and Behavior. 2014 Jul; 4(4): 580–594.

Allen, G., et al. Attentional Activation of the Cerebellum Independent of Motor Involvement. *Science*. 1997 Mar 28; 275 (5308): 1940-3.

Anticevic, A., et al. The role of default network deactivation in cognition and disease Trends in Cognitive Sciences, 16 (2012), pp. 584-592.

Aron, Elaine, Ph.D. The Highly Sensitive Person. Broadway Books; 1996.

Asperger, H. (1991). 'Autistic psychopathology' in childhood. In U. Frith (Ed. & Trans.), Autism and Asperger syndrome. Cambridge, England: Cambridge University Press. (Original work published 1944).

Boss, B. "Autistic?" September 30, 2014. Retrieved from https://www.solvelearningdisabilities.com/tag/add. February 2018.

Beduna, et al. Relationships Among Emotional and Intellectual Overexcitability, Emotional IQ, and Subjective Well-Being. Pages 24-31 | 19 Jan 2016.

Beduna, et al. "Emotions, Cognitions, and Well-Being. The Role of Perfectionism, Emotional Overexcitability and Emotion Regulation." *Sage Journals*, 2015.

Brown, et al. "Sensory processing disorder in mental health." *Occupational Therapy News*. 2006: 28–29.

Bush, G. Attention-Deficit/Hyperactivity Disorder and Attention Networks. Neuropsychopharmacology. 2010 Jan; 35(1): 278–300.

Chang, et al. "Overexcitabilities: Empirical studies and application." *Learning and Individual Differences*. November, 2012.

Chang, et al. "Autism and Sensory Processing Disorders: Shared White Matter Disruption in Sensory Pathways but Divergent Connectivity in Social-Emotional Pathways". PLOS ONE. October 2017.

Clark, et al. Common polygenic risk for autism spectrum disorder (ASD) is associated with cognitive ability in the general population. *Molecular Psychiatry*, 2016.

Coplan, et al. The relationship between intelligence and anxiety: An association with subcortical white matter metabolism. Frontiers in Evolutionary Neuroscience, 3 (2012), pp. 1-7.

Damoiseaux, et al. Consistent resting-state networks across healthy subjects. PNAS September 12, 2006.

De Boeck, (2010, July 15). Brain Functions. Retrieved from http://www.staalhemel.com/2010/brain-functions. January, 2018.

Depping, et al. Abnormal cerebellar volume in acute and remitted major depression. *Progress in Neuropsychopharmacology, Biology and Psychiatry.* 2016 Nov 3;71:97-102.

Edwards, Allison. Why Smart Kids Worry. Source Books; 2013.

Engel-Yeger, et al. The relationship between sensory processing patterns and sleep quality in healthy adults. *Canadian Journal of Occupational Therapy.* 2012.

Epstein, et al. Failure to segregate emotional processing from cognitive and sensorimotor processing in major depression. *Journal of Psychiatric Research.* September, 2011.

Gard, et al. Potential self-regulatory mechanisms of yoga for psychological health. Frontiers of Human Neuroscience. September, 2014; 8: 770.

Green, et al. Salience Network Connectivity in Autism Is Related to Brain and Behavioral Markers of Sensory Overresponsivity. *Journal American Academy of Child Adolescent Psychiatry.* 2016 Jul; 55(7): 618–626.e1.

Hawkins, Jeff and Blakeslee, Sandra. On Intelligence. Times Books, 2004.

He, et al. Scalp Acupuncture Treatment Protocol for Anxiety Disorders: A Case Report. Global Advances in Health and Medicine. 2014 Jul; 3(4): 35–39.

Hofmann SG, et al. The effect of mindfulness-based therapy on anxiety and depression: A meta-analytic review. *Journal of Consulting and Clinical Psychology.* 2010 Apr;78(2):169-83

HSP hsperson.com. https://hsperson.com/faq/spd-vs-sps/ (accessed January 15, 2018).

Immordino-Yang, et al. Correlations between social-emotional feelings and anterior insula activity are independent from visceral states but influenced by culture. *Frontiers in Human Neuroscience.* 2014 Sep 16; 8:728.

Jung, Carl. Modern Man in Search of a Soul. Routledge Press; 1933.

Jung, Carl. Psychological Types; Routledge Press; 1973. (Original work published in 1923).

Kagan, et al. The long shadow of temperament. The Belknap Press of Harvard University Press Cambridge, 2004.

Kanner, L. Autistic disturbances of affective contact. Nervous Child: *Journal of Psychopathology, Psychotherapy, Mental Hygiene, and Guidance of the Child.* September, 1943.

Karpinski, R., et al. High intelligence: A risk factor for psychological and physiological overexcitabilities. *Science Direct.* September 2017.

Kinnealey, et al. "Relationships Between Sensory Modulation and Social Supports and Health-Related Quality of Life". *American Journal of Occupational Therapy*. 2011 May-Jun;65(3):320-7.

Leibowitz, (2017, December 28). Have a High IQ? You Might Be Prone to Physical and Mental Illness, Says Science. Retrieved from https://www.inc.com/glenn-leibowitz/have-a-high-iq-you-might-be-prone-to-mental-physical-illness-says-science.html. February, 2018.

Markram, H., Markram. K, The intense world theory—A unifying theory of the neurobiology of autism. Frontiers in Human Neuroscience, 4 (2010), pp. 1-29, 10.3389.

Melillo, Robert. Disconnected Kids. Penguin Books; 2009.

Melillo, Robert. https://www.brainbalancecenters.com/our-program/integrated-approach/sensory-motor/ (accessed August 29, 2018).

Mendaglio, Sal. Dabrowski's Theory of Positive Disintegration, Great Potential Press, 2008.

Nakao T, et al. Gray matter volume abnormalities in ADHD: voxel-based meta-analysis exploring the effects of age and stimulant medication. American Journal of Psychiatry. 2011;168:1154–63.

Nardi, Dario. Neuroscience of Personality: Brain Savvy Insights for All Types of People. Radiance House; 2011.

Owen, et al. Abnormal white matter microstructure in children with sensory processing disorders. Neuroimage, 2013; 2: 844–853.

Panksepp, et al. The Affective Core of the Self: A Neuro-Archetypical Perspective on the Foundations of Human (and Animal) Subjectivity. *Frontiers of Psychology.* 01 September, 2017.

Penney, et al. Intelligence and emotional disorders: Is the worrying and ruminating mind a more intelligent mind? Personality and Individual Differences, 74 (2015), pp. 90-93.

Ryman SG, et al. Sex differences in the relationship between white matter connectivity and creativity. Neuroimage. 2014 Nov 1;101:380-9.

Siegel, Daniel M.D, Hartzell, Mary M.Ed., Parenting from the Inside Out. Penguin Books, 2003.

Van Den Heuval, et al. Rich-club organization of the human connectome. *Journal of Neuroscience.* 2011 Nov 2;31(44):15775-86.

Van Elst, L.T. et al. Magnetic resonance spectroscopy comparing adults with high functioning autism and above average IQ. Molecular Psychiatry, 19 (2014), p. 1251, 10.1038/mp.2014.160.

Velázquez, J.L. et al. Information gain in the brain's resting state: A new perspective on autism Frontiers in Neuroinformatics, 7 (2013), pp. 1-10, 10.3389/fninf.2013.00037.

Voss, Angie, OTR. The Gifted and Sensory Connection. Retrieved from http://asensorylife.com/the-gifted-and-sensory-connection.html. March, 2018.

www.ingramcontent.com/pod-product-compliance
Lightning Source LLC
Chambersburg PA
CBHW071601220526
45469CB00003B/1086